CW01572427

LOSE WEIGHT

WEIGHT

for life

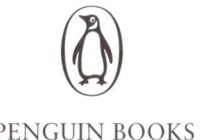

PENGUIN BOOKS

PENGUIN BOOKS
Published by the Penguin Group
Penguin Group (NZ), 67 Apollo Drive, Rosedale,
Auckland 0632, New Zealand (a division of Pearson New Zealand Ltd)
Penguin Group (USA) Inc., 375 Hudson Street,
New York, New York 10014, USA
Penguin Group (Canada), 90 Eglinton Avenue East, Suite 700, Toronto,
Ontario, M4P 2Y3, Canada (a division of Pearson Penguin Canada Inc.)
Penguin Books Ltd, 80 Strand, London, WC2R 0RL, England
Penguin Ireland, 25 St Stephen's Green,
Dublin 2, Ireland (a division of Penguin Books Ltd)
Penguin Group (Australia), 707 Collins Street, Melbourne,
Victoria 3008, Australia (a division of Pearson Australia Group Pty Ltd)
Penguin Books India Pvt Ltd, 11, Community Centre,
Panchsheel Park, New Delhi – 110 017, India
Penguin Books (South Africa) (Pty) Ltd, Block D, Rosebank Office Park,
181 Jan Smuts Avenue, Parktown North, Gauteng 2193, South Africa
Penguin Books Ltd, Registered Offices: 80 Strand, London, WC2R 0RL, England

First published by Penguin Group (NZ), 2013
3 5 7 9 10 8 6 4 2

Copyright © Claire Turnbull, 2013

The right of Claire Turnbull to be identified as the author of this work in terms of
section 96 of the Copyright Act 1994 is hereby asserted.

Designed, illustrated and typeset by Jenny Haslimeier, © Penguin Group (NZ)
Photography by Emma Bass (cover, pages 4, 9, 19, 28, 47, 92, 93, 103,
109, 112, 131, 144, 159, 161, 196, 217–62)
Images by iStockphoto.com (pages 14, 57, 62, 65, 67, 68, 69, 171
and note paper on page 21 and elsewhere)
Prepress by Image Centre Ltd
Printed in China by South China Printing Company

All rights reserved. Without limiting the rights under copyright reserved above,
no part of this publication may be reproduced, stored in or introduced into a retrieval
system, or transmitted, in any form or by any means (electronic, mechanical,
photocopying, recording or otherwise), without the prior written permission of
both the copyright owner and the above publisher of this book.

ISBN 978-0-143-56863-6

A catalogue record for this book is available
from the National Library of New Zealand.

www.penguin.co.nz

LOSE WEIGHT
for *life*

Ditch dieting & lighten up with NZ nutrition expert
Claire Turnbull

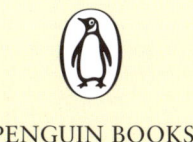

PENGUIN BOOKS

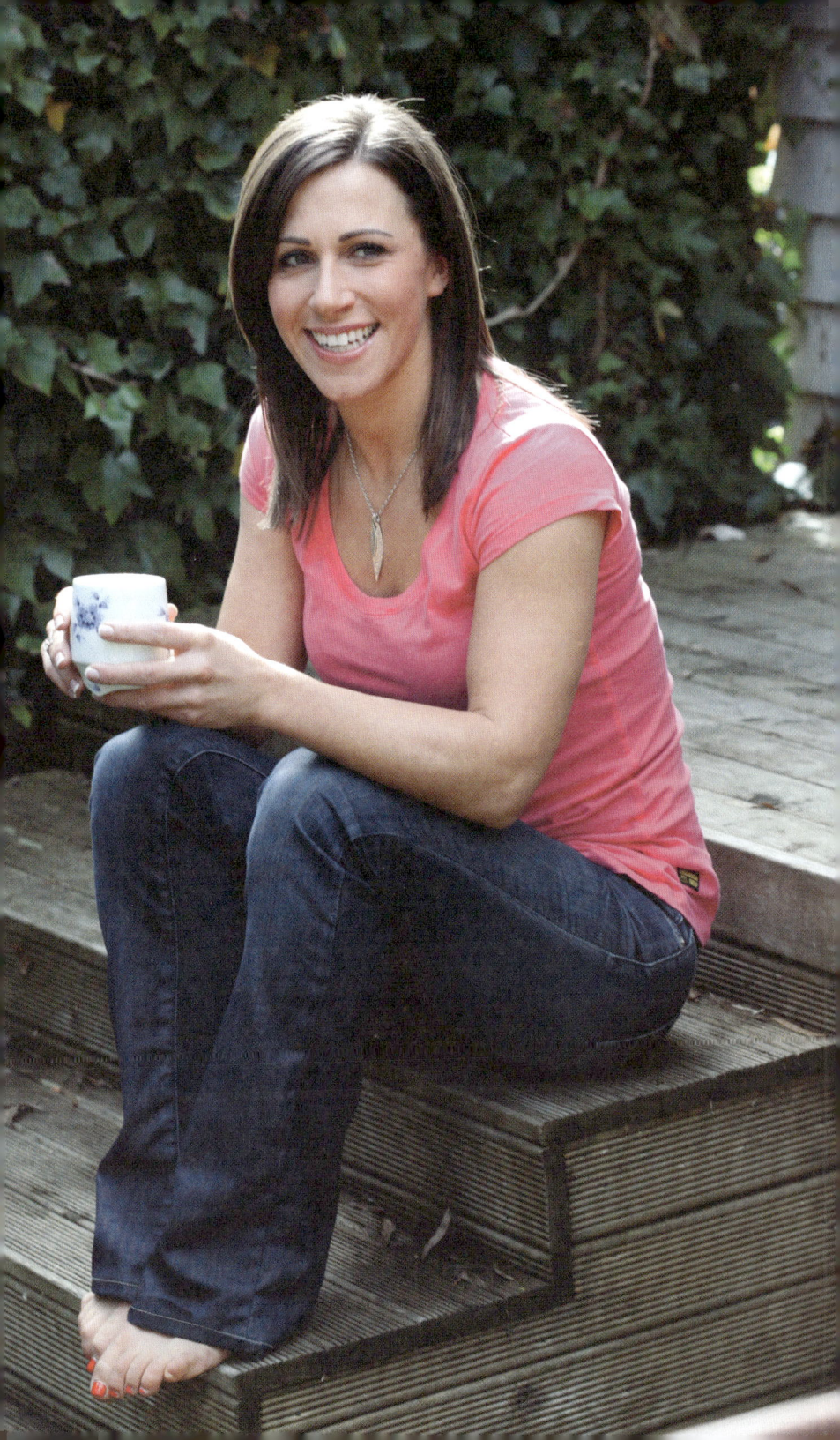

Contents

Foreword

New Zealand, along with every other developed country in the world and many developing countries, is facing a health crisis. We now have a situation where it is more common to be overweight than it is to be a healthy weight, and lifestyle-related diseases, including Type 2 diabetes, heart disease and many cancers, continue to dominate mortality and morbidity statistics. There is no doubt that the way we are eating is at the heart of the problem.

On top of the health crisis, we should also not underestimate the huge impact that food and drink can have on the way we think, the way we feel and how well we are able to function day to day. What people are choosing to put into their bodies these days is less than ideal in so many cases. Claire's excellent book could not be timelier and is much needed when it comes to addressing the problems we face.

While most people realise that their food choices have an impact on both their weight and their health, there is just so much confusion over the best way to eat. A huge part of this confusion has been brought about by the huge array of popular books and magazine articles with fad diets and quick-fix solutions. Freedom of speech is fantastic to allow expression of ideas; but in the case of a science such as nutrition, unfortunately it has meant that it is difficult for the public to assess where the information is coming from and to filter the good information from the bad. It is absolutely essential that solid, science-based nutrition and lifestyle medicine is used as the basis to truly turn our health statistics around. The public deserves and desperately needs good information from a reputable source.

Claire trained in the UK as a dietitian and has expertise in nutrition, exercise and the practical application of lifestyle change. In this book she brings together this knowledge in a highly readable, easy-to-understand but engaging way which I have no doubt will help you to truly understand what you need to do and how to put it into practice. She really does understand that so many people feel like they know what they 'need' to do when it comes to eating, but still, for many reasons, can't do it.

Her own early struggles with her eating and body image give Claire an empathetic viewpoint that not all nutrition experts share, and it is this aspect of the book that makes it stand apart. It's all very well knowing what to eat, but if you lack the tools to change the way you think about food and your body, you'll fail. The practical tips alongside the scientific evidence make this an essential handbook for anyone striving to lose weight and/or better his or her health. I highly recommend it and congratulate Claire on a fantastic, much-needed book.

Dr Joanna McMillan
Dietitian & Vice-President of the Australian Lifestyle Medicine Association
www.drjoanna.com.au

About Claire

I studied dietetics for four years in the UK and have worked in nutrition for another nine years on top of that. I spend pretty much all of my time (sometimes too much time!) talking about, reading about and up-skilling myself in the area of nutrition and wellness. It is my absolute passion.

I am also a huge fitness fan. I trained as a fitness instructor and personal trainer in the UK and, despite not having the time to train others one-on-one anymore, I live a very healthy, balanced and active life myself – it keeps me sane and fit, inside and out.

In truth, though, what I have learnt the conventional way about health and wellness is only part of it. What really fuels my passion for finding long-term solutions to getting people's nutrition and eating habits on track is my personal experience. I spent most of my childhood, teenage years and early twenties being plagued by a very troubled relationship with food. Practically as soon as I started eating, I realised that food could be so much more than just food. It can control the way you think and feel, it can control your weight and size, and other people's emotions when you eat too much or refuse to eat. It can make a day seem good or bad and can make you feel like a success or failure. It has always fascinated me that something as simple as food has such massive power over the way people think and feel about themselves and that something so fantastic can be tied up with so much pain and irritation.

Having worked on my own struggles, I really, truly understand what it is like to know what you need to do but not be able to do it! I know EXACTLY what it is like when food has power over you, because it nearly destroyed and ended my life. Now, with the work that I do and by putting pen to paper, I am passionately striving to help other people break free from the frustrations around eating and go back to enjoying food for what it is – just food!

In my time working in the health and wellness industry so far, not only have I worked with people who know only the basics of nutrition, but I have also helped professionals, such as nutritionists and personal trainers, who really know their stuff but still struggle to apply what they know. In some cases, I have figured out that the more you know, the worse it is. There are so many people who know so much about eating well, but they still have a very dysfunctional, unhealthy relationship with what they eat. Without disclosing any industry secrets, don't assume that because someone looks fit and healthy that they truly are.

Enjoy reading this book and getting your health and wellbeing in great shape! Also be sure to check out my website and Facebook page for on-going hints, tips and ideas.

www.claireturnbull.co.nz
www.facebook.com/claireturnbullnz

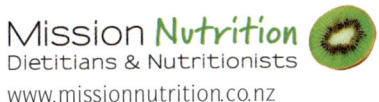

Mission **Nutrition**
Dietitians & Nutritionists
www.missionnutrition.co.nz

Introduction

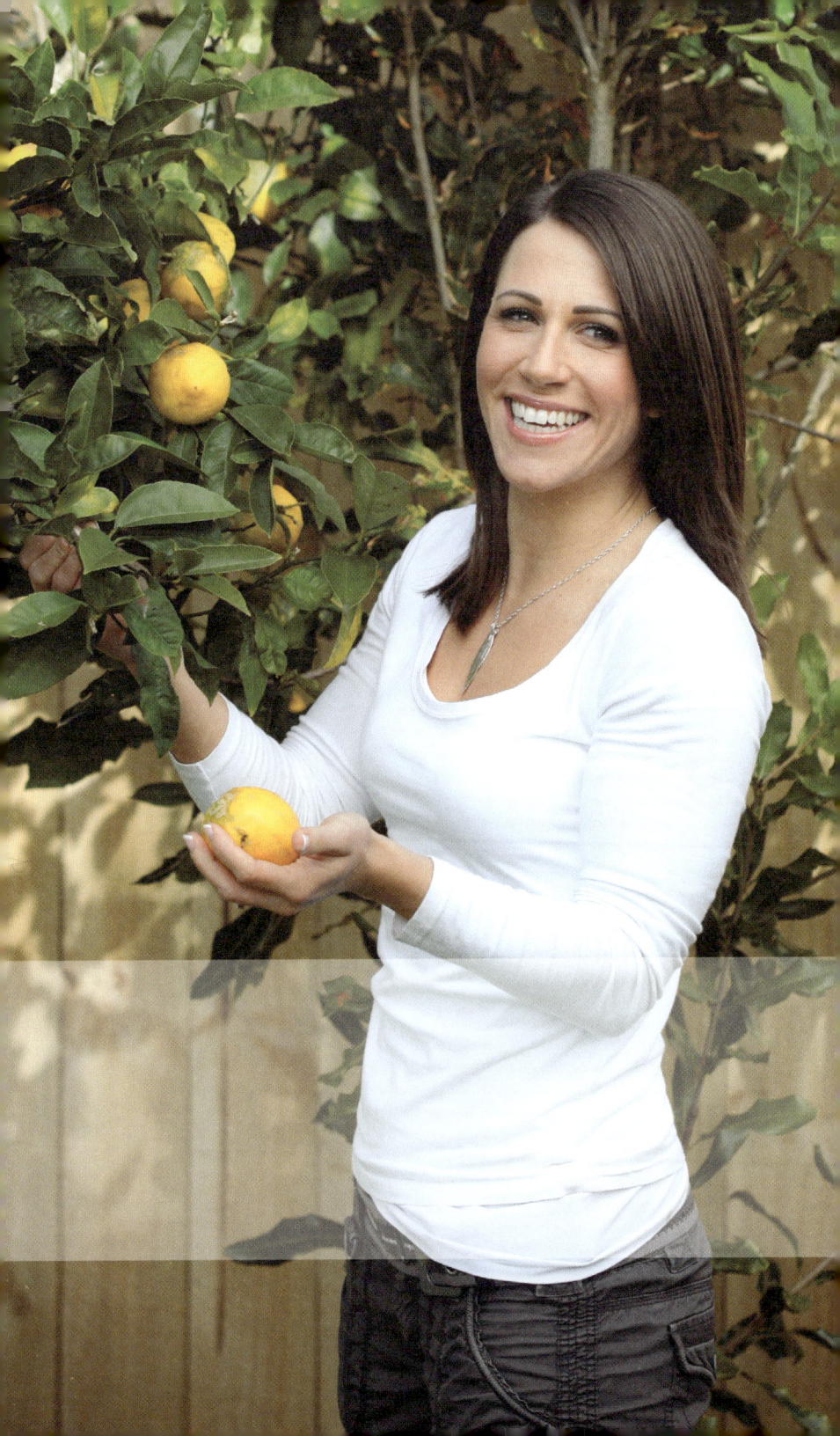

Have you been on a million diets and still feel no healthier? Lost and regained weight a hundred times? Feel like you know what you need to do to get in shape but just can't do it?

If this sounds like you, boy, are you reading the right book! If you are sick of going round in circles and want to make some changes to your health and wellness that will stick with you, read on . . .

Knowing what to do isn't enough

It will be no surprise to you that, as a nutritionist, I spend most of my days (and nights) thinking, talking and reading about food and nutrition. I speak with friends, family, clients, groups, teams and in workplaces. Also, I often get accosted at dinner parties and grilled about my thoughts on various aspects of food and nutrition.

Amongst the hundreds or thousands of conversations, there are a handful of things that always come up, like: 'Is it okay to eat carbs?' and 'How do I shift those last few kilos?' However, there is one thing in particular that comes up every single day from someone, somewhere, and this particular question has become my passion and has led me to write this book. So, what is the question?

'Claire, I have tried so many things to get my eating and nutrition on track, lose weight and keep it off and I really feel like I know what I need to do, but I just can't seem to do it and stick at it. What am I doing wrong?'

We get so many people calling us at Mission Nutrition (my nutrition clinic) saying a similar thing. They have tried everything and are just OVER it! They are looking for a solution that works and lasts.

Barbara is a perfect example of someone in this situation; here is an email we received from her:

Subject: Mission Nutrition – HELP

I need your help. I feel like I know everything there is to know about nutrition, I understand calories, I realise fitness is a big part of getting results, but somehow, for some reason, I struggle with pulling it all together, which is really annoying as I should know what to do. I sometimes overeat and find that food controls me rather than the other way round, which just seems ridiculous – PLEASE can you help!

The truth for Barbara, as for the rest of us, is that just because we know something, it doesn't mean we can apply it to our lives. Yes, I know this seems to defy logic, but that's part of the human condition.

We know that alcohol gives us a hangover and we know how bad that can feel, but often this doesn't stop us from having that fourth glass of wine or eighth beer if we are having fun. We know that eating a packet of Tim Tams after a terrible day at work will provide only temporary pain relief and that afterwards we are likely to feel guilt, self-hatred and disappointment. Still, we eat the biscuits.

Of course, knowing what to eat, understanding nutrition, and being clear on what constitutes a healthy balanced diet is very important (and I will be sharing everything you need to know about that in Section Three) but it's vital to note that just because you know something doesn't mean that you can or will do it! Knowledge alone does not get you what you really want.

> ## Knowledge
> What you know about eating well, exercise
> and keeping healthy

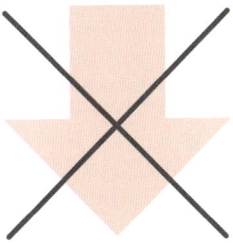

> ## The desired outcome – what you really want
> Happy with weight, size and feeling fit and healthy

SO, WHAT'S THE ANSWER TO ACHIEVING YOUR GOALS AND GETTING RESULTS THAT LAST?

If learning all about nutrition, calories, portions, vitamins and minerals doesn't necessarily get you the results you are hoping for, then what is the answer? I asked this very question of a group I was talking to a few weeks ago in a gym, and here were their responses:

Jane: People just need more willpower.
Ben: I reckon people need to be weighed every week and be accountable to someone.
Theo: It is best when someone tells you off when you haven't eaten as you should have done so you know not to do it again.
Hannah: I would enter a 12-week challenge to get focused.

Do these sound like things you would say or you have heard before? On the surface, they sound very logical and in the short term may get you results, help you to lose weight and get your nutrition on track – but, if you are reading this book you have probably tried to do these things before. Did they really work?

If you have tried to get healthy and lose weight before, I have no doubt that, at some point, you will have had those internal conversations about 'trying harder', 'being more focused', 'doing better tomorrow' – but you know as well as I do that they make very little difference in the long run. When you try to make changes to the way you eat, old habits can replay themselves, and even after completing a '12-week challenge' or being 'weighed in and accountable' to someone for a while, within a few weeks, months or years of finishing the programme, you are very likely to be right back where you started.

So, why is that? Well, it is because none of these approaches provide the answers to making changes that last. In fact, I would go as far as to say that some of these things will fuel the cycle of failure and, for some people, lead to disappointment and self-destruction.

Beating yourself up, negative talk and being angry with yourself for not having applied what you 'know' can lead to a dysfunctional relationship with food and, in some cases, a brutal cycle of emotional eating. Having to be 'told off' by someone, needing to be weighed and judged, will only work for as long as you see this person in authority. Ultimately, the only person to who you need to be accountable is YOURSELF and if you never learn that skill, you are unlikely to get to where you want to be. As for 12-week challenges, they vary in quality and some may indeed be a good way to get you focused, but the notion that your health and wellness has a start and a finish date, in itself, sets you up for failure. I don't need to tell you how many people revert back to their original ways of eating and drinking when these challenges are over – let's just say, lots. So, there must be a better way!

MAKING CHANGES THAT LAST

There are hundreds of reasons why we might want to make changes to the way we do things. It might be that we want to change the way we work, the way we act in relationships, the way we cope with stress or, as we are discussing here, the way we eat

When it comes to making changes on the food front, in my experience there are often three main reasons why people just can't do it, even when they know what they need to do. These reasons have very little to do with willpower or not being good enough. For some people, all these things have impacted on previous attempts to lose weight. For others of you, it might only be one or two of these things.

1. **Deeply embedded eating habits and behaviours** that are your 'default mode', which hold you back from making changes that last. This is addressing things like picking at food, eating when you are bored, not planning meals and so on. To make changes

to these habits and behaviours requires time, practice and reprogramming the way you do things.

2. **Changes to routine or challenging times arrive,** and any plans, good intentions or healthy habits go right out the window! Holidays, weekends, stressful times and any change to your normal routine can send you into a frenzy.

3. **An emotional or dysfunctional relationship with food.** This is when, quite frankly, food messes with your mind. Maybe you end up sabotaging your own efforts (eating a tub of ice cream all at once because you didn't go to the gym in the morning and are now mad at yourself) or maybe you feel that food controls you (you think about it all the time) and you have a love/hate relationship with what you eat.

WHAT'S STOPPING YOU?

This diagram demonstrates that knowledge is not directly linked to outcome. It shows you that there are a whole heap of STEPS in the way to work through before you can make a change that lasts.

Knowledge
What you know about eating well, exercise and keeping healthy

Habits/ behaviours	Challenging times	Food messing with your mind
Your normal food routine	Managing when things change or get hard	Emotional eating
Planning	No time	Self-sabotage
Cooking	Work days	Eating for comfort
Healthy shopping	Busy days	Eating for punishment
Portion control	Holidays	
	Stressful times	

The desired outcome – what you really want
Happy with weight, size and feeling fit and healthy

GETTING TO WHERE YOU WANT TO GO

Now, don't get me wrong, knowing what to eat and when to eat it is still a very important part of the process in helping you lose weight, and we will be looking at this more in Section Three, but the difference with the Lose Weight for Life approach is the application of this knowledge – that is, dealing with the habits and routines, overcoming challenges and managing emotions around food. In doing these things, you will have a road map to achieving your wildest dreams! The Lose Weight for Life approach helps you overcome the barriers that have previously stopped you from getting results and, even more importantly in my view, maintaining them. After all, it's not that hard to lose weight; it's keeping it off that's the challenge.

Here's the normal weight-loss pattern for about 95 per cent of people:

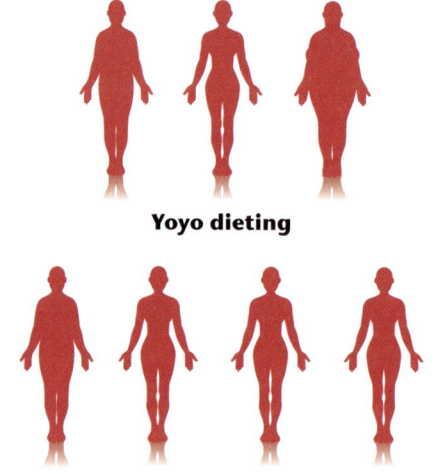

Yoyo dieting

THE LOSE WEIGHT FOR LIFE APPROACH

YOUR HABITS AND BEHAVIOURS LET YOU DOWN AND THINGS CAN GET CHALLENGING

As human beings we are creatures of habit and when we learn to do something a certain way it can be VERY hard to unlearn it. This principle absolutely applies to the way that we eat. Although it may seem logical to want to eat more healthily, drink less alcohol and exercise more, the outcome of your 'want' will depend not only on what you learn about the topic (kilojoules, serving sizes and so on), but also on the habits and behaviours you have to permanently alter to get the outcome you want.

To eat more healthily, you have to shop more healthily, cook more healthily and monitor your portions – so far, so good. But what about when you get busy? What about when your routine changes? You start a new job? You go on holiday? It comes to the weekend? Conceptually, it is pretty straightforward to eat well (more good stuff, less junk), but to actually eat well (and by that I mean balanced, not eating only lettuce) 365 days a year, you need to be able to cope when things get tough, not just on a quiet week at work or when the kids are being well behaved!

People often seem to wait for a good time to change the way they eat, a good time to start cooking healthy meals . . . but like cleaning out the garage, painting the front room or getting round to planting a herb garden, there is never a good time. Now, right now, is as good as it is going to get. Making changes to the way you do things is a journey, a process, and ideally should have a positive, lasting impact on your life.

HAS FOOD MESSED WITH YOUR MIND?

For some people, food is just food. It fills a gap and eating is something they do simply to live. For the rest of us, this is so far from the reality. Despite knowing that food is essentially 'just food' and that bread or cake can't bite us or talk to us, somehow food can still mess with our minds and make us feel quite uneasy. It can control how we feel about ourselves! How odd is that? It's just food, isn't it?

For most people, eating is about enjoyment, taste and sharing, but in our society it can also be used as a reward and as a punishment. Along the way, from the situations and experiences in their lives, for some people food has acquired an additional meaning and, in some cases, food can actually end up controlling them.

Feeling guilty after eating, sabotaging your weight-loss efforts by eating cake in private when you are angry at yourself, skipping meals to try to lose weight and then bingeing later on, hitting the booze when you walk in the door from work to help get rid of the stresses and pressures of the day – these are all examples of using food to do something that it was never designed to do. If this sounds like you, no amount of learning about the concepts of 'good nutrition' will help you reach your desired outcome. You need to deal with the situations and circumstances around food first.

But panic not . . . that is why I am here and, in the coming sections, I will work with you to help you overcome these obstacles so that you can Lose Weight for Life. To break the cycle and get results, the answer is changing or, more precisely, transforming your food habits and behaviours at the same time as dealing with your thoughts and feelings about food. I aim to show you how to work on all three parts of the diagram on page 13.

Getting the results you want is not about following a nutrition plan for a set number of days or going in to be weighed week after week, but instead is about creating long-term healthy habits and behaviours which will allow you to eat and apply what you know about eating well to your life, every day. It is also about being able to overcome challenging days, busy times and any emotional connection that you have with food.

From here, all you need to do is forgive yourself for any unsuccessful previous attempts, acknowledge the things you have learnt and enjoy this moment right now . . . because, from here, anything is possible. I can't wait to show you how.

THE LOSE WEIGHT FOR LIFE APPROACH

- Is NOT a 'diet'
- Can work for everyone
- Helps you to get results that LAST
- Sorts out the facts from the fiction when it comes to nutrition
- Helps you design your own eating plan
- Helps you plan, cook and eat healthy meals
- Looks at your habits and eating behaviours
- Helps break the cycle of emotional eating.

Most weight-loss plans and diet programmes address only the 'knowledge' side of things. You may end up with a list of what to eat and what not to eat, which can work for a while – but, as you know, this approach doesn't get to the root of the problem and, sadly, it is unlikely that these plans and programmes will help you long term. That is where the Lose Weight for Life approach is different, helping you to understand the reasons why you are carrying more weight than you want and finding tailor-made solutions just for you.

How? I will help you come up with the answers.

The other failing in weight-loss programmes is that often they do not encourage you to take responsibility for yourself and you end up being accountable to someone else with endless weigh-ins and meetings where you are told off for eating cake and overindulging. That might sound like what you need (and most people think it is), but again, it really doesn't help you get to where you need to go! In the following pages I will help you to become responsible for yourself and deal with the reasons why you are eating more than you want or need to and the times when you may be sabotaging your own success. Throughout the book there are exercises which encourage you to think about why you are the way you are, and why you eat the way you do. You will need a pen and paper to write things down as we go, so find yourself a nice notebook to scribble in, or write directly on the spaces provided in the book. It is VERY important to take the time to stop and do these exercises, so don't skip them!

WHAT YOU WILL GET FROM THIS BOOK

The Lose Weight for Life approach is about changing the way you eat, losing weight and keeping it off, using a combination of my knowledge, professional and personal experience, and it is an approach that can work for everyone. Here is a summary of what we are going to be covering:

1: Getting Started – understand yourself and set your vision for the future

- Understand who you are and why you think the way you do.
- Gain insight into your relationship with food.
- Clarify how your thoughts, beliefs and emotions are influencing your food choices.

- Identify the challenges you face in your current environment.
- Learn to accept who you are.
- Focus on what it is that you really need to be working on to Lose Weight for Life.
- Understand change and how to make changes that last.
- Set a vision and goals.
- Use what has happened in the past to help you now.
- Set up support to help with your journey.
- Get your mind in the right space.
- Measure your success.

2: What You Really Need To Know

- Make sure you know who to listen to.
- Eat what your body needs.
- Be clear on serving sizes so you can Lose Weight for Life.
- Understand your digestive system.
- Learn what choices are best within each food group.
- Know how to keep well hydrated.
- Understand how exercise can help you reach your goals.
- Know the power of quality sleep.

3: Making Things Happen

- Keep your vision at the top of your mind.
- Make sure your nutrition, exercise and wellbeing knowledge is up to scratch and clear up any confusion.
- Create your own healthy habits and routines.
- Cope with challenging times.
- Manage when food has messed with your mind.

4: Can't-fail Quick-and-easy Recipes

- Brilliant breakfasts
- Lively lunches
- Fabulous main meals
- Nutrition information for sides
- Snacks and sweet treats

I hope that you find in these pages a fresh approach to help you make long-term changes to the way you eat and overcome the challenges that have held you back from getting lasting results. Now it is my turn to help you, so tune in – let's see what's going on for you! Things are going to get interesting . . .

1

Getting Started

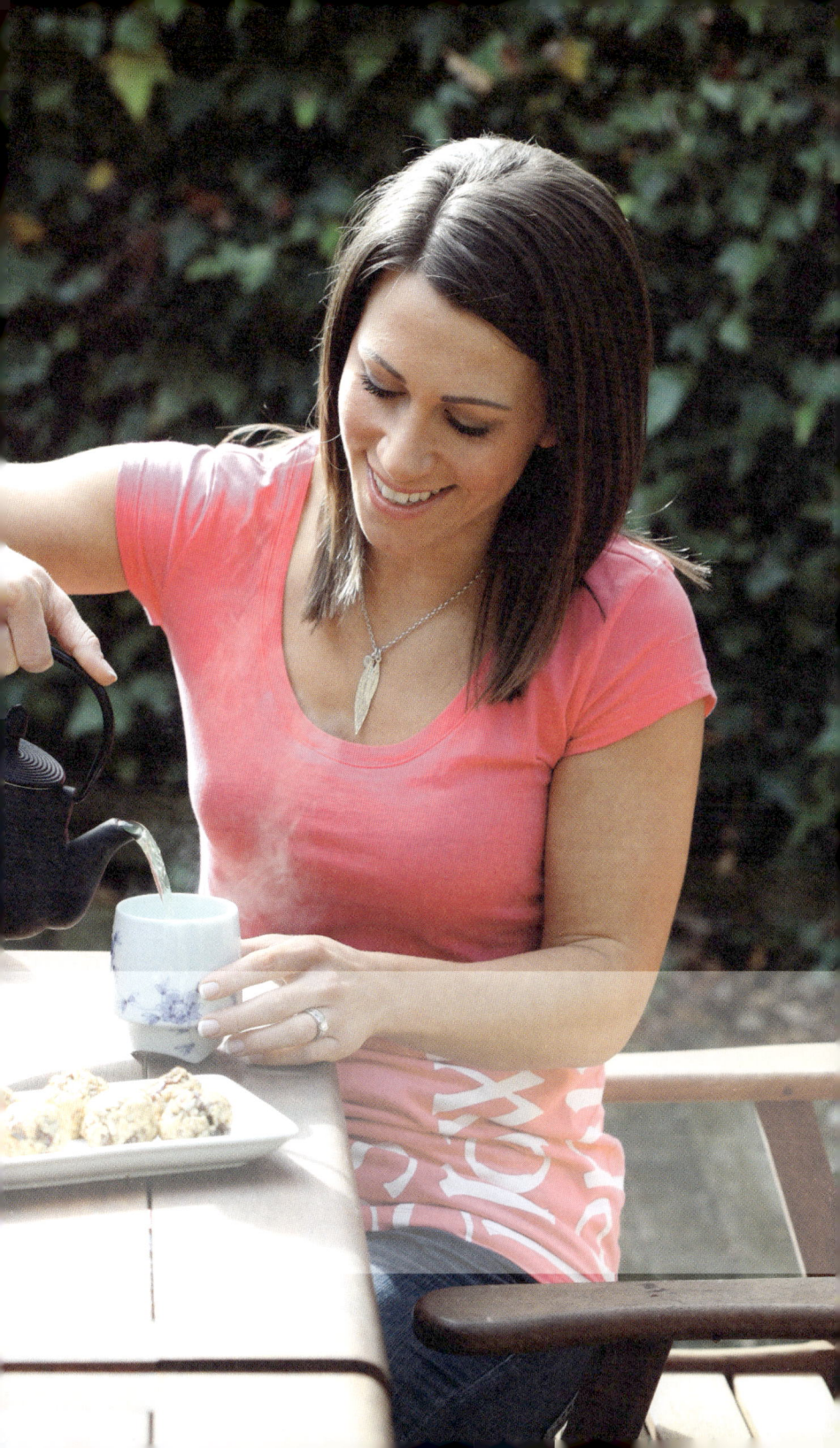

This is such an exciting time. You are embarking on a journey which will not only help you to lose weight and keep it off, but will also help you to learn a lot more about yourself, which is important in so many ways.

To get started we will be looking at where you are at right now, what your life looks like, how you think and feel about food and what things from the past have impacted on the way you eat today. You will then be able to identify what you really need to work on to get the results you deserve, at the same time as building a better relationship with the essence of who you really are.

I will be helping you to understand the process of 'change' and showing you why sometimes even though we know things (like what we need to eat to lose weight), we just can't or don't do them.

It is then time to create a vision, set some goals and make sure you have a plan in place to support your changes. So, let's get into it!

Part 1: Where are you at RIGHT NOW?

Making permanent, positive changes to the way you eat will allow you to get the results you are looking for and Lose Weight for Life. Unlike other weight-loss programmes where the first steps are to jump on the scales, set yourself a mega goal and quickly start some kind of semi-starvation diet, the Lose Weight for Life approach focuses first of all on *you* – who you are, why you eat the way you do and what food really means to you. Why? Well, because without being very clear about where you are at RIGHT NOW and WHY, it is very difficult to make changes that last.

FOOD AND YOU

I could write a whole book on the reasons why 'diets' don't work, but essentially what it boils down to is that following a set plan of exactly what to eat, trying to restrict your food intake to unrealistic amounts or ban certain foods altogether doesn't deal with the root cause of you carrying more weight than you want to. Diets are band-aid solutions which may temporarily get results and help you to lose weight, and they may even work for a year or so. However, the truth is that as soon as your situation changes – you come up against a rough patch in your life or a difficult day – you are likely to go back to the way you used to eat or sabotage your best efforts by bingeing, going off your diet or just giving up on trying to eat well because it is all too hard.

To get results, lose weight and KEEP IT OFF requires changing the way you do things at a much deeper level – that is, changing your whole approach to food and your relationship with it.

Your habits and behaviours

Some of us feel the need to lick our plates clean before leaving the table, others of us nibble on biscuits when we are bored, and there are those of us who eat at a hundred miles an hour. The habits and behaviours we form, both in our childhood and as adults, are incredibly important to understand, particularly because it is often these habits and behaviours which lead us to overeat or make unhealthy food choices when we really don't want to.

YOU TIME: Let's look at your habits and behaviours

Get out a pen and paper (or, alternatively, write in the spaces provided below) and take some time to think about the following questions. Jot down everything that comes into your head. This is not a time for you to judge right or wrong; it is just a chance to look at the facts of your life to see if you can identify things which may be affecting the way you do things now. Your list of notes will really help you when it comes to finding out what you need to be working on to lose weight and we will be referring back to them later.

1. Do you always have to finish everything on your plate?

2. Do you pick at food and nibble rather than eating meals and snacks?

3. When it comes to meals, do you plan what to have for the week or just work out what to eat one day at a time?

4. Do you eat at roughly regular times or is it really erratic?

5. In the morning, do you always pick up a coffee or feel you need a coffee to start your day?

6. When you do your food shopping, do you check the labels of what you are buying?

7. Do you find it hard to say no to alcohol when others are drinking?

8. How much oil do you use when you are cooking? Do you pour mindlessly or only use a splash or a spray?

9. When it comes to portions, do you have any idea whether you eat the right amount for your body? Do you think you maybe eat too much?

10. When things get busy, do you get takeaways or just skip meals altogether?

The list of questions I could ask here is endless, so just think for a minute now about any other habits you have when it comes to food and things which affect the way you eat, what types of food you eat and how much you eat. Write as many notes as you can. The clearer you can be on your current situation, the easier it will be to work out what changes need to be made.

_____

_____

_____

_____

_____

_____

_____

_____

_____

_____

_____

_____

Your environment and its challenges

Think for a moment about someone you have met who lives a totally different life to you. Maybe you were brought up in a busy city and they were brought up on a farm. It could be that you are an only child and they have six brothers and sisters. They may have different types of friends to you or different beliefs about the world and the way things should be run.

Whether you are aware of this or not, the environment in which you were brought up, be it the school you went to, the size of your kitchen or how close the nearest supermarket was to your home, will have had an impact not only on the person you are today but also on the way you eat and your relationship with food.

The same goes for your current environment: where you work, the friends you spend time with and the places where you go on holiday – these things all play a part in the way you eat.

Understanding your environment, past and present, along with your habits and behaviours, will help clarify why you do the things you do and why you may shop, cook and eat in a certain way.

When you have a clear understanding of who you are, you will be in a position to effect change, to make choices about your life, to head in the direction where you really want to go, and, as part of that picture, to lose weight and keep it off without having to go on another hideous diet!

Many people believe that life just happens to you and that you have no control over where your life goes, but that really couldn't be further from the truth. Regardless of your past, where you come from and what you have been through, when you are able to accept who you are you will be able to make choices about everything you think and do, and this has a profound effect on where you can go in the world.

YOU TIME: What was your environment like growing up? And now?

Again, without attaching meaning, just jot down everything you can for each of these questions. Some of these may overlap with the answers from the previous questions, but that doesn't matter. Get all your thoughts, feelings and emotions out on paper, allowing yourself to be very clear on what you currently do when it comes to food.

1. How many people lived with you when you were growing up?

2. Did you sit down and eat as a family?

3. Did you eat in front of the TV?

4. Did you serve yourself at dinner or was your portion served up for you?

5. If you have siblings, did they have any impact on the way you ate? Did you have to eat quickly to make sure you got a chance to have seconds if you wanted them? Did you finish the leftovers on anyone else's plate?

6. Did you learn to cook as a child?

7. Were you involved in making food choices? Did you ever help plan meals?

8. Did you get involved with food shopping?

9. Was your family on a tight food budget? Or could you afford to buy whatever you liked?

10. Did you take food to school from home? Or did you buy lunch at school or on the way there?

Next, it's time to think about your environment right now. Think about what is going on in your life at the moment. Answer the questions overleaf and see if this leads you to understand more about why you eat or drink the way you do. Again, no judgement here; this is not about feeling bad about the things you do, just about understanding yourself and seeing things as they really are.

1. Is your life really very busy? Do you find that a lack of time holds you back from eating well?

2. Is eating well at work a challenge?

3. If you are at home most of the day, do you pick, nibble or find it difficult to establish a good eating routine?

4. Do you have to eat out as part of your job? Is drinking wine and networking part of your normal working day?

5. Does your current routine involve heading to a café most days? Having morning and afternoon tea out?

6. Is there high-fat, high-sugar food readily available all the time at work or in your house?

7. Does it always seem to be someone's birthday? A reason to have a slice of cake, have a drink to celebrate (or commiserate) something, or endless parties you just *have* to attend?

8. Does your social life revolve around food and drink?

9. Do you use alcohol to help you relax, cope with stress or unwind?

10. When you go on holiday, do you leave all your healthy habits behind? Eat and drink anything you want?

Your thoughts, beliefs and emotions

Did someone call you fat when you were a child or tease you about your weight? Was someone in your family on a diet, always trying to lose weight? Were sweet foods used as a reward for good behaviour?

At certain points in your life, be it a traumatic event, someone saying something really hurtful or you seeing someone doing something you didn't like, for a number of different reasons single moments such as these can become very significant. Whatever it was and however it happened, what you need to know is that for all of us there will have been several important points in our lives when, unconsciously, we will have formed 'beliefs' about certain things. In some cases, these beliefs will be around food, weight and how we look. As well, some people will have learnt to use food or drink to help manage an emotional feeling, be it for comfort or, in some cases, as punishment and self-sabotage.

Let's look at a few examples of this.

Samantha put on quite a lot of weight in her early teenage years and other kids at school started to tease her. She ended up feeling like she had no one to talk to and no real friends. She ate more to comfort herself and, in a way, to punish herself for how she was. From the things which were said to her and the experiences she went through at school, at some point she created an unconscious belief which embedded itself deep into her mind: if she was overweight she wouldn't be able to have friends or ever be loved.

Twenty years later, without her really being aware of it, this belief still controls her thinking. Even though as an adult she now has great friends who enjoy her company, deep down she has huge insecurities when it comes to relationships because part of her believes she can't be loved. Even though she is now slim most of the time (her weight goes up and down), she is so scared of putting on weight that she has a really disordered relationship with food, goes from diet to diet and finds it difficult to get close to men as subconsciously she believes they won't love her if she ever gains weight.

For Samantha, no detox diets, food diaries or daily weighing will help her get what she really wants: a healthy relationship with herself and food, being a stable, healthy weight and shape and having meaningful relationships with other people. For Samantha, to overcome her challenges and Lose Weight for Life, she needs to work on what she believes and reprogramme that part of herself.

John is another person who has been through it all when it comes to food. When he was younger his parents used to fight all the time, and I mean really fight. They threw things, yelled and screamed and it always ended up in tears. John used to sit upstairs in his bedroom crying, feeling so scared and helpless that he couldn't do anything to make the fighting stop. He felt so incredibly alone. Always, though, after a fight his mum would eventually come upstairs and sit on the end of his bed and tell him she was sorry. To make him feel better, she would bring him biscuits, chocolate or cake and tell him that he was just to enjoy them and not worry about anything.

From the time John was four years old he believed that food wasn't just fuel; it was something that could be used to change the way he felt and thought about a situation. Ever since, he has used food for things that it was never designed for – to control emotion, ease pain and provide comfort. John is now very overweight, binges in private after bad days at the office and has huge guilt because he realises that he uses food to comfort his own children when something goes wrong in their day.

For you, this may be an area which needs very little attention or it may be an area which needs a lot of work. If there are any underlying beliefs which you have around food, we will need to address them to allow you to move on because, with this stuff happening in the background, regardless of how much you 'know' or 'learn' or 'conceptually understand' about nutrition, you will be unable to make significant changes to the things you do around food which come from your unconscious beliefs. We will be finding a solution to this later on pages 198–215.

YOU TIME: Your experiences and beliefs

Time to hit your pen and paper again. As always, scribble down as much as you possibly can.

Think about any significant events, circumstances or situations in your life which might have led you to create certain beliefs around food. What happened? How did you feel? What did you make the situation mean? What do you now do because of this experience? Has it changed the way you think and feel about food?

Here are some examples of things that you might do now because of certain experiences you may have had and beliefs you have formed.

- Eating food for comfort when you are sad.
- Eating a huge portion of food when you are angry at yourself.
- Feeling like you've failed if you eat one chocolate or a single biscuit when you're on a diet. You carry on eating because you have 'blown it' so might as well keep going.

Great. By now you probably have a little book or a few pages (or hundreds of pages) which are all about you! It doesn't have to all make sense yet; this is just a really good starting point and platform to work from. All will become clear later on.

My story

I was brought up in the north of England. I went to an all-girls school, have two brothers and my mum was always on a 'diet' for as long as I can remember. Every single detail of my life, my environment, my experiences and the habits I learnt along the way all affected my relationship with food and my beliefs around it.

At school, there was a massive focus on what you looked like. Girls started dieting from the first day I rocked up there, aged 11, and it was a never-ending cycle of skipping meals to keep slim and bingeing on chocolate at sleepovers.

My two brothers hugely impacted on my relationship with food. At mealtimes, I would serve myself as much as possible to start with as I knew there would never be second helpings and, if there were, the boys would have polished them off before I got a look-in.

Then there is my mum, dieting her whole life. I guess that made it normal for me to see someone weighing their food, eating different things to everyone else and controlling the amount they ate to make the number on the scales head in the right direction.

I could give you a million more examples of even the most minor things in my life which have affected how I think and feel about food: the speed at which I learnt to eat, the amount I thought was normal to put on my plate, using food as comfort in times of sadness and starving myself to get attention. Despite what people may look like on the outside, most people, particularly women, will have been through some similar things to me; some less so, some more so, but for many of us, food at some stage has come to be more than just fuel.

This is your journey and, in the same way that my life has affected my beliefs about food, yours will have too. It is exactly these experiences that you need to be aware of to be able to move forward and overcome all the things which have held you back from losing weight and keeping it off. The future is bright and yours for the taking.

Your relationship with food

You may wonder why I asked you to write lots of notes about yourself and your life. Well, I would like you now to take a moment to look back at what you have written. Look at your life and look at the role food plays. Are there particular habits, thoughts, beliefs or experiences which are part of the reason that you are struggling with your weight today? Is it everything you have written down, or just particular parts? Get a highlighter pen, go back through what you have written and figure out what are the biggest things in your life that you think have had an impact on your weight and wellness today.

The reason I am asking you to do this is not so you can call up an old school friend and have a go at them for suggesting that you were the 'chubby one', or to start hating your mum for making you finish everything on your plate or giving you chocolate when you were sad. That will get you nowhere. In fact, it is likely to do the opposite and send you into a 'victim state' where you can't move forward because you are holding on to hate, resentment and blame.

Instead, I want you to see things exactly as they are, to understand a little more about yourself and see clearly that to move forward, lose weight and keep it off, you will need to make peace with some of the things which have happened to you in the past, as well as address unhelpful thoughts and beliefs about food and find solutions to any habits which have resulted in you using food for something it wasn't designed to do.

The list and notes that you have jotted down will be unique to you, and your starting point for doing things differently, having a healthy relationship with food and losing weight for life.

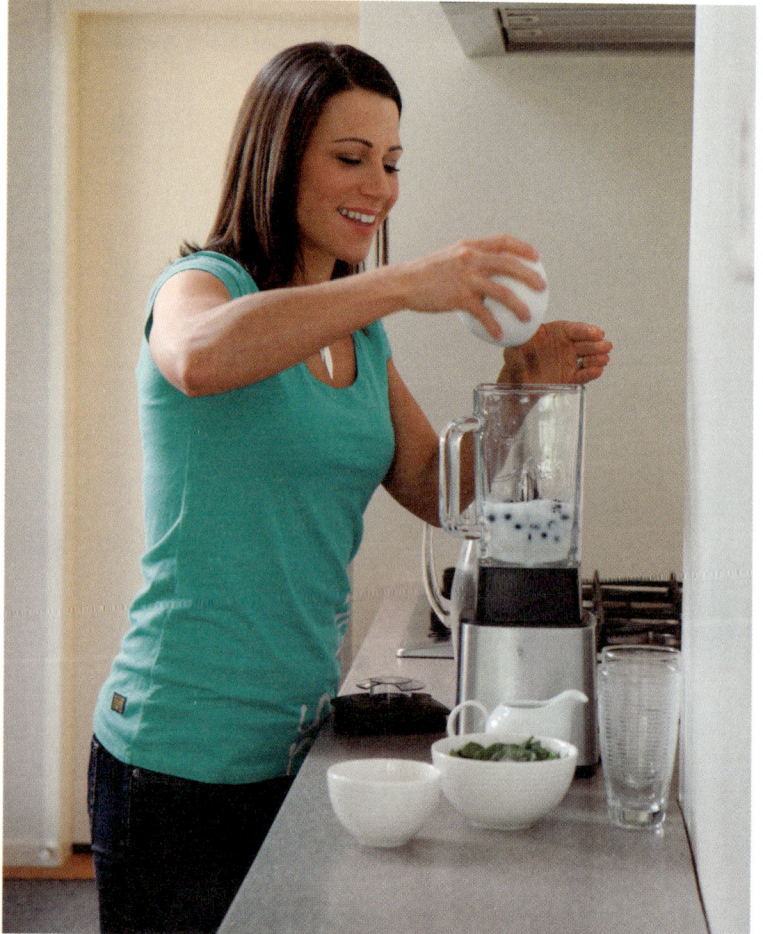

NOW YOU KNOW YOURSELF BETTER — WHAT NEXT?

Looking at your life exactly as it is can be pretty tough. To go back over hurtful times and difficult situations isn't always easy, but it is worth it because when you can see things exactly as they are, you will have the choice about what to do next. To Lose Weight for Life, here is what you need to do with what you have learnt about yourself:

1. Give up any excuses.
2. REALLY accept who you are.
3. Work on things that can be changed:
   - Get your knowledge right.
   - Address unhelpful habits and routines.
   - Find solutions for challenging times.
   - Manage your mind when it comes to food.

1. Give up any excuses

Be responsible for yourself. This is your time to shine.

We are all full of excuses. When it comes to losing weight, I must have heard them all. Whether it is that you are too busy, you were bullied for being overweight or have to eat out for your job so can't lose weight — let's be honest, these are all excuses.

I don't mean to be harsh or blunt, but I guess, in part, I need to be, because as long as you are using an excuse, however big or small, the only person who loses out is you.

If you can reflect back on your lists, answers and experiences, there will be things that have happened to you in the past, things people have said and done and reasons why, to this point, you have not been able to lose weight and keep it off.

As hard as it is, the brutal truth you have to face right here, right now, is that as long as you use these excuses, you won't be able to Lose Weight for Life — you will be held back by things in your past.

A few years ago, I read and learnt a lot about the concept of 100 per cent self-responsibility, and it was an incredible thing. I always thought that I was responsible for myself but, as with everybody, there were a whole heap of excuses that I was carrying around, based on my past, to explain why I couldn't do certain things in my life. Coming through the other side and seeing that being responsible for yourself, forgiving others for things they have done and said and giving up excuses which don't serve you is liberating and exciting, and an essential step to creating the life you really want.

So, without getting too deep and meaningful on you, take some time to think about the excuses you use and that you will need to give up, remembering that if you don't do this, it is only you who loses.

YOU TIME: What excuses do you use for not being able to lose weight or eat well, which you need to give up?

_____
_____
_____
_____
_____
_____
_____
_____
_____
_____
_____
_____
_____
_____

2. REALLY *accept who you are*

You are the only you; you are unique and that is awesome. The goal, I guess, is to be the best you – and that is not about fixing or changing who you are, but more about accepting all parts of yourself. When you are okay with who you are, you can move on to working on (not fixing) the parts of yourself, your habits, behaviours and beliefs, the things you have learnt in your journey through life, and allow them to work in your favour, work to help you reach your goals, rather than working against you.

I can honestly confess I spent the first 20-plus years of my life wanting to be someone different. I thought that other people somehow seemed to be able to do things better than me, they looked better and they were happier than I was. How wrong I was. If you spend all your life focusing on the things you don't like about yourself and trying to be someone else, you just end up going round in circles and, over time, hating who you are and being disappointed in yourself because, in some way, you feel like you aren't good enough.

I have come to understand that being happy is about being okay with who you are and accepting all the good things about yourself, as well as being okay with your flaws. If you aren't able to accept what you are and what you're not, you will never be able to find real peace in your life or reach your goals and dreams. An important step in being able to break free from the dieting cycles and negative feelings about your weight and size is to, right here, right now, stop fighting with yourself, stop hating yourself for what you aren't and accept that you are human and have a combination of good and not-so-good traits.

Here is a quote I just totally love:

Be yourself, everyone else is taken.
Oscar Wilde

You are unique

The way you look, the way you think and the way you do things is completely unique, and what a fabulous thing to celebrate – life would be so incredibly dull if we were all the same.

When it comes to the way we look, there are some things about ourselves that we can't change such as our ethnicity, our height and, without hideously painful surgery, our eye colour. Some of us are more likely to gain weight around the middle, others will have naturally chunky thighs and then there are the more fortunate ones who find it super easy to keep slim.

As much as we would like to get into the cells of our bodies to swap our DNA for the mix of genes we really want, that is just not the way it is and, in my belief, not the way it should be – there is something beautiful about being able to accept who you are.

Now, I am not suggesting you give up caring about what you look like and say goodbye to your hairbrush and favourite clothes. There are some fabulous things we can do to make the most of ourselves, such as using make-up, plucking our eyebrows and having wonky, unruly teeth straightened, but my message is this: please don't be under the illusion that independently these things will make you happy. They can certainly make you feel better about yourself, but my belief is that true happiness and peace comes from a much deeper place and has very little to do with the colour of your hair or the size of your thighs.

In my life, I have met so many people who are beautiful in so many ways but they still spend an inordinate amount of time, money and energy trying to fight their genetic make-up and change massive things about who they are. In most cases, they are no happier in the end.

My advice is to do whatever it takes to be at peace with yourself and love who are you from the inside out. From this point you will come to realise what really matters in the world and that, despite all your flaws, you are best to make the most of what you have rather than spend your whole life trying to be someone different.

YOU TIME: Are you really okay with who you are? What parts of yourself do you need to learn to accept? Write them down.

_____
_____
_____
_____
_____
_____
_____
_____
_____
_____
_____
_____

3. Work on things that can be changed

Accepting yourself is one thing, but to lose weight and keep it off there are some things in your environment, as well as some of your habits, behaviours and beliefs, which can be worked on, and this is what I will help you do throughout the following sections of this book.

Look at your notes and then tick all the things below which you feel you need to address in order to lose weight and keep it off. Add anything else you have identified from your writing, too.

- [ ] Brushing up on nutrition knowledge.
- [ ] Meal planning.
- [ ] Healthy food shopping.
- [ ] Healthy cooking.
- [ ] Addressing portion sizes.
- [ ] Avoiding eating or picking at food just because it is there.
- [ ] Eating better at work.
- [ ] Managing social times, especially when alcohol is involved.
- [ ] Eating better on holidays and trips.
- [ ] Giving up excuses.
- [ ] Working on accepting yourself for who you are.
- [ ] Overcoming a dysfunctional relationship with food.
- [ ] Managing emotional eating.

Other:

_____
_____
_____
_____
_____
_____
_____
_____
_____
_____
_____
_____
_____
_____
_____
_____
_____
_____

The rest of the book is structured to help you work on each of these things one by one – hurray, it's action time!

Making changes

Now that you have a better understanding of who you are and some of the challenges you face, it's time to think about how you can use what you have learnt about yourself to start making changes and getting the results you are looking for.

ALL ABOUT CHANGE

Change is the most interesting thing. There are some changes which we are very happy to embrace which are nothing but super exciting. Getting a pay rise at work, the arrival of your first child or decorating your bedroom to make it everything you have ever dreamed about – beautiful and fabulous! Other changes are a total nightmare and seem to bring nothing but drama, negative emotion and terror – stopping smoking, having the courage to leave an unhappy relationship and, of course, embarking on a weight-loss journey. I can feel your blood pressure rising just thinking about these changes. Not a nice feeling, is it?

The truth is, as I am sure you will have heard before, there are three things which are absolutely certain in the world: one, your life will eventually come to an end (sorry, a sad start but it does get better); two, you need to pay taxes (in most countries); and three, THINGS CHANGE.

As difficult as change can sometimes be, it really is a good thing in most cases, either because it can make your situation better or you learn something about yourself along the way which helps you to grow and develop as a person.

There is an unbelievable number of different perspectives, philosophies and ideas on change. Visit any online book store and you will find hundreds of thousands of books on the topic. There are books written by psychologists, anthropologists, scientists, leadership experts – the list is endless, really. If you want something in your life to change, my belief is that it boils down to looking once again at three things. First, you need to CHANGE THE WAY YOU THINK; second, you need to CHANGE THE WAY YOU DO THINGS; and last, you need to CHANGE YOUR ENVIRONMENT to support the changes that you want to maintain.

Commonly, when people embark on a weight-loss journey they will only work on one or two of these things, not all three. For example, if you know that part of your weight issue is that you drink too much wine, you can DO something differently by making yourself a green tea when you walk in the door from work – that is a fabulous start and most of the time this might work for you.

But . . . what happens at the weekend when you catch up with your friends? Can you resist getting stuck into the wine then? It is not that you need to stop going out and never touch alcohol again, but if you want to make long-term changes to your weight THAT LAST, you may need to alter your environment, too, when it comes to alcohol or whatever area it is that you need to work on.

As an alternative to always meeting your friends for a drink, why not sometimes think about catching up and chatting while out on a walk together, over a cup of tea, or doing some activity not revolving around alcohol – particularly if this is a common occurrence for you and part of what is taking you away from your long-term goal?

If you use alcohol to cope with stress or as your default to unwind when you walk in the door, you may need to find a solution to this, too. In part, this might be working on changing the way you think. If your default thought when you walk through the door is: 'I have had a hideous day, all I need is a wine to help me relax and I deserve it', before you know it, all good intentions aside, you will have a wine in your hand and end up feeling annoyed at yourself for going against your goal to drink less. It is fine for you to have that default thought, but you have a choice whether to listen to it or not; and you can also have a new thought you can plant in your head when you walk through the door – for example: 'I have had a hideous day, I could have a wine to help me relax, but I know this is taking me away from what I really want, so I will call my friend for a chat to cheer me up instead.'

Whatever the challenges you need to overcome to lose weight, be it portion control, exercising more or healthier cooking, you are likely to need to address this on many levels: changing what you THINK, changing what you DO and changing your ENVIRONMENT to support the changes you need to make. Another thing to consider is that, as fabulous as it is to find someone else to make you accountable for your actions, someone to insist you count kilojoules or write down everything you eat, as I have alluded to before, ultimately it is important to be accountable to *yourself*. If you don't learn these skills, as soon as you stop 'checking in' you can quickly slip back to your old ways. At my nutrition clinic, Mission Nutrition, we offer one-on-one nutrition support, coaching and guidance which works very well, but ultimately our goal is not to have people come to us every week of their lives and confess what they have or haven't eaten; instead, our goal is to help people to be responsible for themselves long term and to make changes which last.

I know this approach may all sound far harder than the cabbage soup diet or counting points, but really it is just a step-by-step journey and one that is so incredibly worthwhile. After all, what is the point of embarking on this project to Lose Weight for Life if you can't keep up the positive changes you make?

In the coming sections I will be guiding you through step-by-step ways to change how you THINK about things, how you DO things and how to change your ENVIRONMENT to ensure that whatever is holding you back from losing weight and keeping it off is a thing of the past. Power to you – it is time for change, time to put YOU in the driving seat of your life and wellbeing.

WHAT DO YOU ACTUALLY NEED TO CHANGE?

When you consider change, it is interesting that sometimes what you need to alter isn't what you might first think. What do I mean by this? Well, let's look at an example.

Ann is a 45-year-old lawyer who has always struggled with her weight. From looking at the way she eats, how she thinks and feels about food, she identifies that she eats too many biscuits at work. The biscuits sit in a large jar in the shared kitchen where she works and every time she goes to make a cup of tea, she sees them and has one or two. So, she recognises this habit needs to change to help her get in shape.

She comes up with the plan of taking an apple every day and having that instead of the biscuits, a logical approach. Problem is, she gets bored eating apples very quickly, sometimes she forgets them and sometimes she ends up picking at the biscuits just because they are there.

Really, by bringing an apple, she has only solved part of her problem. To successfully beat her biscuit habit she also needs to look at altering her evironment. She could put the biscuits in the cupboard so they are out of sight and less tempting. She could also ask if the biscuits could be replaced with fruit, and put out for people to see. Alternatively, she could go to the second kitchen in the building, which has no biscuits, or she could put a kettle in her office and have her tea in there, being sure she takes a break at some point during the day to get out of her office. As well as changing her habits and environment, she also needs to look at how she thinks.

This is only one example, but it highlights that sometimes the solution which comes to mind first isn't always the best one. If you want to eat less, it is not just about serving up less on your plate. It is also about cooking less to start with and buying less at the supermarket. So what might seem like a portion-control issue is actually more to do with being able to write a good shopping list and buying no more than you need to cook.

If you binge on chocolate or ice cream when you are feeling down and upset with yourself, the logical thing might be to not have these foods in the house (even though you can go and buy them on your way home if you really want). Really, though, the thing you might need to change here is how you cope with your emotions and the way you think and feel about yourself. Do that, and you might not even need to banish the foods you enjoy as they won't have the power over you that they once had.

YOU TIME: What do you ACTUALLY need to change?

Using your list from page 32, which identifies what you need to work on, think for a moment about what you ACTUALLY need to change – is it what you do, the way you think, your environment, or all three? Write some notes.

_____
_____
_____

ARE YOU REALLY READY TO CHANGE?

I understand that this seems like the most ridiculous question, as you have got as far as reading this book; therefore, it would seem pretty logical that you want to change. However, I ask this question for a very important reason – as human beings, we often don't like change and even if in our minds we really want to do something, there may be deep, dark emotional stuff going on which means that, although on the surface you want to lose 10 kilograms, some small part of you doesn't. If that part isn't dealt with, it can win the fight and stop you from losing weight.

To explain this almost ridiculous concept, let's meet Mary.

Mary was 38 at the time I met her. She had a fabulous job as a director of a marketing company, loved being busy, loved socialising, loved wine and parties, but had gained 10 kilograms in the last few years and wanted to feel fab in her clothes again and get rid of the extra rolls which had arrived without warning.

When I first met Mary, on the surface it seemed impossible to think that she was anything other than 110 per cent ready to change. She was sick of her clothes being tight; she was sick of feeling fat and told me she would do anything to get rid of the weight! Anything? Umm . . . we will see! So, after setting Mary off on a plan, helping her establish healthy eating habits and routines, plan meals, work out which alcoholic drinks were the best low-kilojoule options and what to prepare at the weekend when friends came over, in one of our meetings it struck me like lightning: deep down, Mary didn't want to change. In fact, this part of her was absolutely committed to NOT changing. I know that sounds absurd, but she was having real issues with something which Debbie Ford (a very well-respected American lifestyle coach and author) describes as 'underlying commitments' or an unconscious agenda. Deep down, Mary was more committed to being 'popular' and 'liked' than she was to losing weight. As a result, her underlying commitment was winning; she couldn't make changes because part of her didn't want to.

Jenny Devine, a fabulous leadership coach right here in New Zealand (www.jennydevine.co.nz), introduced me to Debbie Ford's work and, in her book, *The Right Questions*, she describes underlying commitments as being 'responsible for the discrepancy between what we say we want and what we're actually experiencing' (p.43).

Let's look at some other examples of how these 'underlying commitments' can play out:

- You declare that you desperately want to be slim and yet you continually snack on chocolate bars. When you ask yourself what you are truly committed to, you find that it's making yourself feel good in the moment or instant gratification. You want pleasure NOW and truthfully that is what you are really committed to – more than being slim.

- You constantly compare yourself with images of slim, beautiful women in the media and state that is how you want to look. But no sooner do you begin a weight-loss programme than you beat yourself up for being unattractive and hopeless. You ask yourself, 'What am I most committed to?' and you realise that it's feeling bad about yourself. Playing the role of 'the victim' is what you are most committed to – net result, you don't change.
- You tell your friends and family that you want to lose weight so you can attract your perfect partner and in public you eat the 'perfect' diet – healthy salads and low-kilojoule drinks – but, as soon as you get home, you eat the fatty, sugary comfort food you love. When you reflect deeply on why you do this, you realise that being overweight makes you feel safe from male attention and advances.
- You work with a nutrition specialist to come up with the 'perfect' diet and exercise plan for you and then choose to watch TV instead of exercising. You eat whatever food takes your fancy. You remember that, as a child, your parents were extremely controlling and you realise that your deepest commitment is to be a free spirit: 'I'll do whatever I want, whenever I want.'
- You are gregarious and love to socialise. Eating out and drinking alcohol is part of the fun for you. You know the weight is becoming more and more of an issue but you keep putting off doing anything about it. When you ask yourself what is the cause of the procrastination, you understand that you are committed to being liked by people as a fun party girl and any change to that would risk you becoming boring and less popular.
- You have a healthy eating guide and a great exercise regimen to follow, but you keep changing them and are determined to make them more suitable for you and your lifestyle. Subsequently the weight doesn't shift. You notice that despite working with the most knowledgeable health and fitness people in the business, you're most committed to 'doing it my way'.

Being aware of any underlying commitments that you may have is a great first step. Look back on the notes you have written so far. Can you see any such underlying commitments or any conflict between what you want and what you are currently doing? You might find that even though part of you REALLY wants to change, another part of you really wants to stay the same!

But fear not: once you have identified any underlying commitments, you have the power to choose to do something about them and address them. The aim is to create a new set of commitments that are more in line with your vision, goals and dreams. So, what is getting in the way of you getting where you REALLY want to be in your life?

Part 2: Where EXACTLY do you want to be?

After looking in detail at who you are, why you eat and exploring the concept of change, the exciting part has now arrived where we put together a road map for you with specific instructions to help you get started on your weight-loss journey.

DOING THINGS DIFFERENTLY THIS TIME

1. Creating a vision

I would like you to think for a minute about what you would really love your life to be like. Shut your eyes and think about how you would look, how you would like to feel when you wake up in the morning. What things that bother you right now would no longer be issues for you? Create a very clear vision in your mind and stick with it for a minute or two. How do you feel? What is it that is so different to the way you are living right now?

Now, write down everything you see, and everything you feel. Part of this may be that in your vision you are wearing smaller clothes. You are fitter and feel more energised. Get real about what it is you are aiming for, the best *you* that you can imagine yourself to be.

_____
_____
_____
_____
_____
_____

Next I want you to write a description of your life in one, two or five years' time (whatever feels right for you) as if you were living the life you most deeply wanted. Where are you? What are you wearing? How often are you exercising? What kind of foods are you eating? How do you feel about yourself? What are you doing every day? How are your relationships? Write in the present tense – it is incredibly powerful for rewiring your brain and thoughts. PLEASE don't skip this; it is one of the most important things you can do. It may feel odd to start with, but it is vital to help you get where you want to go.

_____
_____
_____
_____
_____
_____

As well as writing your thoughts down and being clear about where you want your life to go, collect some pictures of how you would like to look and feel, things that motivate and inspire you. Put them in your note-book, on a board, or somewhere you can see them. Without bursting your dream bubble, be realistic if you can. If you are 157 cm tall and have an hourglass shape, however many pictures or images you collect of someone who is 183 cm tall with a natural pencil-thin figure, that's not really the best YOU, is it? You would need a miracle and a lot of painful surgery to get there.

Got your vision? Good.

2. Setting yourself goals

Okay, now it's time to move from the vision to your goals. How are we going to get you from where you are right now to where you want to be? You can choose as many goals as you like, but my suggestion is that you start with three things you would really like to achieve. Try to make your goals not just about numbers and sizes, such as 'I want to lose 10 kilo-grams and I want to be a size 10', but rather about how you will feel: 'I am feeling comfortable in my clothes' or 'I feel confident when I am wearing togs'. Also, maybe think about a goal related to energy levels, fitness or self-confidence.

You will see here that I am writing these goals in the PRESENT tense! Please do the same – it is critical. For you to reach these goals and get to where you want to be, you have to truly believe in them, integrate them into your being and feel like they are part of you. If it is very difficult to do this, start with 'I wish I was', 'I would like' and 'I should be able to' and so on. Here are some examples of goals you might want to set – all written in the present tense.

- I feel confident in my clothes.
- I am okay with letting my partner see me naked (with the lights on).
- I feel super energetic.
- I fit into clothes which make me feel good.
- I can walk/run 5/10/15 km (or whatever is right for you).
- I can finish an exercise class without feeling like sitting down halfway through.
- I am able to buy clothes from wherever I like, rather than plus-size stores.
- I enjoy food without guilt.
- I don't rely on food to make me feel better after a bad day.
- I stop eating when I feel full.
- I trust myself around food.
- I don't panic when I have to go out for dinner or go to a buffet where I will be surrounded by food.
- I am okay with who I am and don't judge myself.

YOU TIME: What are your top three goals?

1. _____
   _____
2. _____
   _____
3. _____
   _____

Now that you have identified your top three goals, we need to look at these in a bit more detail and be really clear about what it is that you want to achieve. Being specific is vital when you are setting goals, as any vagueness means you will readily come up with excuses to not follow through with your plans. You may not be able to fill all these things in now; that is fine – you can come back to these goals throughout the book and redefine them, tweak them and get clear about what it is that you really need to be doing differently – but it is a great start to work on this now.

For each goal, I would like you to think about these things:

1. What do you need to DO differently to reach your goal? Do you need to shop differently? Cook differently? Eat smaller portions? Are there any unhelpful thoughts you might need to work on? Is there anything in your environment you can change to help make reaching this goal easier?
2. WHEN would you like to have achieved this goal? Put a timeframe on this. Be realistic, and put down a date and time in your diary when you can assess how things are going. This is NOT something for you to use to judge yourself and feel bad if you don't get there on time. It is just a good starting point so you have something to aim for.

GOAL 1:

1. What might you need to change?
   _____
   _____
   _____
   _____
   _____

2. When do you want to reach your goal?
   _____
   _____

GOAL 2:

1. **What might you need to change?**

    _____
    _____
    _____
    _____
    _____

2. **When do you want to reach your goal?**

    _____
    _____

GOAL 3:

1. **What might you need to change?**

    _____
    _____
    _____
    _____
    _____

2. **When do you want to reach your goal?**

    _____
    _____

3. What are the consequences of not reaching your goals?

This is a VITAL STEP in goal setting and vision planning which is so important but easy to miss. It is helpful to have a good think about what it will be like if you don't follow through with your goals. It might be that you stay the way you are and nothing changes. It might be that you continue to gain weight. Whatever it is, write it down and think clearly about what your life will be like if you don't make some changes.

_____
_____
_____
_____
_____
_____
_____
_____

So, why does this matter? Well, the thought of these consequences can help motivate you to stick with your plan, to reach your goals and not give up, and I guess you are reading this book because you want something to change and be different. If everything stays the same, you aren't any better off!

4. What is the reward for following your plan and achieving your goals?

Now, it doesn't matter who you are or where you come from, we all love a reward for hard work. Keeping yourself motivated during any change is really important. There will be times when things are tough, you go off track, it all seems a bit too hard – but when you have a reward in sight, it can make it that little bit easier to get back on track.

The reward you choose needs to be unique to you and preferably nothing to do with food! Maybe you will treat yourself to some new clothes, go away for the weekend or have a holiday. Perhaps it is shouting yourself a massage, spa day or magazine subscription. You may want to choose different rewards for different goals, or one for the whole lot – whatever works for you. Again, write it down; make it real so you are accountable to yourself.

5. What has worked for you in the past?

Think about previous attempts you have made to lose weight and get healthy. What in the past has worked for you and helped you? It might have been writing down what you eat. Or using scales and measuring cups to see how much you were eating. It may be that you were working with someone else or had support from a friend or family member.

Here, I am looking for you to identify positive, HEALTHY things that have helped you before, which you might be able to incorporate now. Counting kilojoules and weighing every scrap of food you ate might have worked, but is not really a long-term solution or a healthy thing to be doing in most cases as it can breed a degree of obsession around food. So avoid writing things down which are not realistic, long-term behaviours. Instead, it might be that using measuring cups and smaller bowls or plates most of the time or menu planning is helpful for you. Have a think and jot things down.

_____
_____
_____
_____
_____

6. What has held you back in the past?

If you have tried to lose weight in the past or change the way you eat, what are the things that have held you back? These are things you will need to be mindful of with your journey, too, and by identifying these things you can work on them and change them so they no longer become issues for you.

So, what has held you back? Work colleagues bringing in junk food? Over-indulging at birthday parties and celebrations? Eating out and not being able to control yourself? Sad days? Being too busy? Get clear . . . and write these things down. You may find you come up with some excuses here, too; which, as you now know, need to be given up – they won't help you.

_____
_____
_____
_____
_____

7. What might get in the way of you reaching your goals this time?

So you have looked at things which have made you fall over in the past. What about now? What are the barriers and triggers you need to be mindful of?

Maybe you have kids and you pick at their food after eating. It could be that your husband, partner or flatmate brings home big bags of chippies on a Friday night and puts them right under your nose. Come on . . . brain time – what is going to get in the way? If you know what the issues may be – you guessed it – you can deal with them!

_____
_____
_____
_____
_____

8. Who is going to help you on your journey?

Now I know I have gone on and ON about self-responsibility, but it can be
very helpful to have someone who is working on this with you or who you can
talk to about things. Maybe it is a friend who has bought this book, too, so
you can work on this together. Maybe it is a friend with whom you share your
hopes and dreams. After reading this book, it may be a nutritionist for some
personalised advice, or a coach, psychologist or counsellor to help you deal
with some of the things that have come up. There is no right or wrong here:
who you choose to support you is up to you, but, be assured, having some
support can only be a good thing.

_____
_____
_____
_____
_____
_____
_____
_____
_____
_____
_____
_____

9. Getting your mind in the right place

Your mind is super powerful and you have the ability to control what you think
and how your life turns out. When things don't work out as you would like or
you have a day when things turn to custard, try not to judge yourself or beat
yourself up – it won't help and will only make things worse. Instead, look at
what has happened during the day as if you were someone else looking in on
your life impartially. What happened? What was going on? This is a journey,
and when things don't go your way it is such a fabulous opportunity to learn
something. So, rather than feeling as though you have failed when things go a
bit pear-shaped, think about what you can take from the situation. How can
you make sure that it doesn't happen again?

10. Be ready to set new goals

Okay, maybe not yet! I know you haven't even started on the ones you have
just written. But be ready to revisit this section of the book any time you like
and rework things, set yourself new goals or redefine them when you have
reached the ones you are working on right now.

MEASURING YOUR SUCCESS AND THE TRUTH ABOUT THE SCALES

When you are on a mission to lose weight, lose body fat or tone up, there is a temptation to get fixated on the scales and define your progress on the numbers alone. In my experience, though, this is just not all that helpful. There are SO many things which can affect the numbers on a day-to-day basis, such as the time of day, how much water you have had, when you last went to the toilet, the clothes you have on, how much exercise you have done and, of course, for us women, the time of the month. There can also be variations between different sets of scales.

The only ideal way to measure someone's weight and body composition is to do something called underwater weighing or by using very expensive machines which scan your body and are able to fairly accurately work out where you are at. This is really only done in labs and at universities, so, for the rest of us, we need to use the tools that we have available to us. These are scales (there are various types, of course), measuring your waist and hips with a tape measure and the changes in the tightness (or hopefully loosening) of your clothes.

My recommendation to people trying to lose weight is to take some baseline measurements at the start (weight, waist and hips) and maybe take a photo of yourself in your togs or underwear. Then weigh and measure yourself no more than once a week and don't start obsessing over every millimetre or gram gained or lost. It is not helpful.

If you are the kind of person who gains 100 grams and feels like a failure and will end up eating 10 chocolate bars for punishment, scales aren't for you. There are other ways to track your progress and some big things you need to work on in terms of the way you think about yourself and food if you want to Lose Weight for Life.

If you do decide to weigh and measure yourself, please track the measurements over time to show a trend. In my mind, these numbers are NOT the only markers of success. The biggest wins will be in how you look and feel.

Part 3: MAKING things happen

To make things happen you need knowledge and skills to help you get on and stay on the right track. In the next sections we will work through everything you need to know and do to be sure you are successful on your weight-loss journey. I will help you set up a healthy eating plan, create healthy habits and routines, overcome challenges and manage your mind – so, let's get into it!

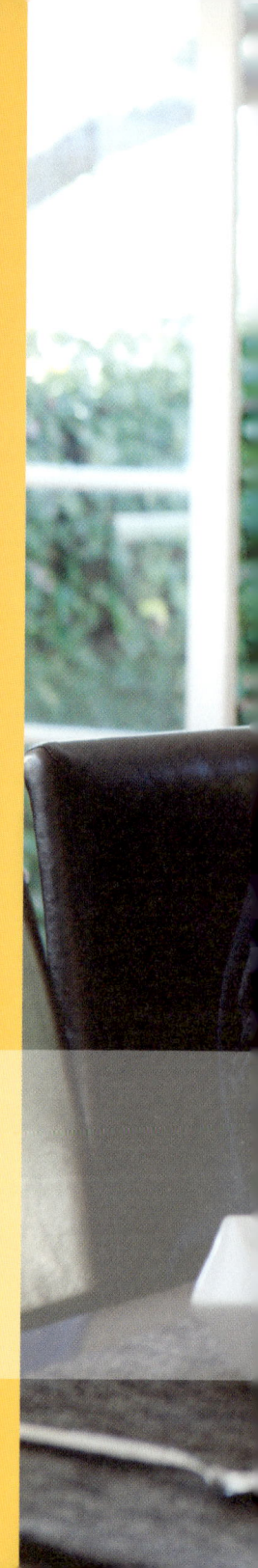

2

What You Really Need To Know

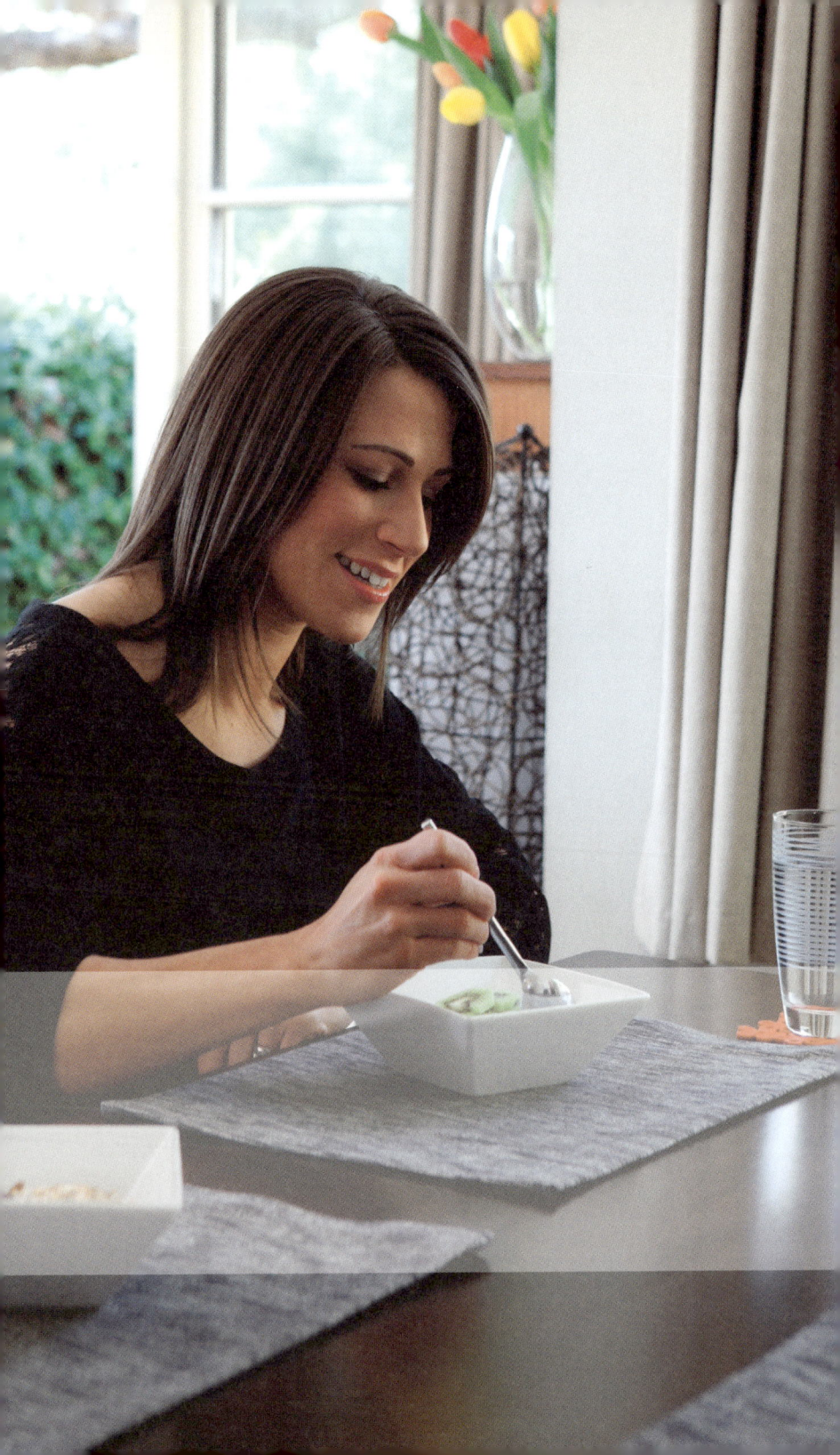

Part 1: Nutrition 101

Now you have set your vision and have your goals all sorted out, let's start the ball rolling on making some changes!

Despite my clear view that knowledge alone is not enough to help you lose weight or to change your eating habits and behaviours, it is still super important to make sure you know your stuff. Having a good base understanding of food and nutrition will give you a very clear picture of what your body needs and why. Then you will know what to aim for when it comes to eating the right balance of foods and making informed choices about what you want to be eating. Another bonus of understanding what the real function of food is and what happens to it after you have eaten it is that it can help you see why fad diets, quick fixes and false-promise diets are only short-term solutions to much bigger issues.

As well as being your guide to what to eat and when, this section of the book explains weight-loss theory, helps you to read food labels and helps you work out how much you need to eat. I will also talk you through the role of sleep and exercise in your journey to Lose Weight for Life.

You will then be able to put together a personalised plan so that you know what you are aiming to eat each day to ensure your body is able to function at its best and that you are optimising your overall health and wellbeing. When you have your plan sorted, the all-important crunch time is next, and this is where I believe the answer to getting lasting results really lies. That is, putting your plan into action and overcoming any unhelpful habits, behaviours and thoughts which will otherwise hold you back – all coming later in the book.

My ultimate goal is to help you get into a good routine with your food and feel that you have the power to choose what you eat, rather than having the feeling that food controls you. I am going to help you overcome the barriers which, to date, have held you back from being the best you. So, let's get cracking and make sure you know your stuff.

WHO TO LISTEN TO WHEN IT COMES TO NUTRITION

Ask three people the same question about nutrition and I bet you will get three different answers. When should you eat your biggest meal of the day? Is it okay to have carbs after 5 p.m.? Are supplements a good idea? With everyone seeming to believe they are an expert in nutrition these days, alongside differing opinions and ideas wherever you look, it can be hard to know who to listen to, what is the best path to take and what ideas are just money-making scams.

What you read in a magazine this week about carbs being 'the devil' will be different from what you read in the same magazine next week about 'healthy carbs being the hidden secret to a red-carpet body'. The same goes for what you see on current-affairs programmes, weight-loss shows and in newspapers. You can even pay to see nutrition experts – dietitian, nutritionist, naturopath – who may tell you very different things. So why are there such contrasting points of views about how food affects you and what you need to eat to be fit and well?

DIFFERENT POINTS OF VIEW

We are all different. We look different, smell different, like to have different hair-styles, wear different clothes and when it comes to solving a problem we might all take a slightly different approach. Whether it's your political point of view, your beliefs about parenting or the best way to iron a shirt – there are many different ways to think about one thing or, as the saying goes, more than one way to skin a cat!

The same goes for health and nutrition. There are endless opinions about the best way to optimise the health of the human body and some of them, just like a good political debate, will end up with people disagreeing when they reveal their very different perspectives.

With nutrition, there are hundreds of different approaches, but rather than using the entire book to debate every approach that can be taken, I will start simply, with the following . . .

The medical minds

In New Zealand, like much of the western world, the approach we have most commonly been exposed to up until recently is an evidence-based approach to health and wellbeing, using research as the basis of decisions made and advice that is given. This is known by some as the medical model. What this means, in real terms, is that before advice is given on a topic, for example eat more fruits and vegetables to help prevent cancer, there has to have been a huge number of very good-quality studies done (experiments, if you like!) to make sure that what you are being told is, to the best of the medical world's knowledge at that point in time, correct. This is traditionally the approach taken by your GP, nurses, hospital doctors, surgeons, physiotherapists, speech and language therapists as well as dietitians. Nutritionists with university degrees will also have been taught in this way and have these beliefs about food. People who work in this area of health are commonly obliged to be registered, undergo regular reviews to ensure the information they provide is up to date and accurate and are mostly required to have some form of insurance cover. In New Zealand, the Ministry of Health guidelines are based on this approach, as is the work of reputable organisations such as the Heart Foundation, Diabetes New Zealand and 5 + A Day, and *Healthy Food Guide* magazine.

The difficulty some people have with this approach is that they see that the advice given can sometimes change over time – such as with eating eggs. In years gone by, people were told not to eat eggs at all if they had high cholesterol, but now the advice is that including a limited number of eggs can be okay. This is because the more up-to-date research now shows that the type of cholesterol in eggs doesn't have the same effect on the cholesterol in the body as researchers used to think it did. So, sure, it can be confusing, but it is important to understand why things change. As we learn more about the world, about food and about the human body, research progresses and we find out things that we didn't know before. That pretty much applies to the rest of the world, too!

For years, throughout the world, smoking was promoted heavily on TV and on billboards, and tobacco companies even sponsored sports events, but in recent years, as we have learnt more about smoking and its effects, the advice has changed.

When I was little it was normal to be told that you MUST eat everything on your plate or you wouldn't get dessert; now we know such an approach can lead to a dysfunctional relationship with food, and alternative ways to encourage children to eat vegetables and healthy, balanced meals are recommended. I can see why people may lose faith in the medical model because of this, but now that you see why things are the way they are it might help remove some distrust. An important thing to remember, though, is that if you choose to disregard science and research, you are only listening to anecdotal evidence and opinion which has its own massive set of problems.

Alternative thoughts

The alternative approaches to health and wellness are far and wide, from traditional Chinese medicine, herbal medicine, homeopathy and naturopathy to yoga therapy. Such approaches are often based on historical or cultural beliefs and traditions rather than specific scientific evidence (as is the base of the medical model). These alternative approaches have been lurking in the background of the western world for many years, but with the increasing fast-paced flow of information and ideas being shared on the internet, alongside people aspiring to be their own 'health expert', the desire for options outside the medical model seems to be growing.

The difficulty with this area is that although there are truly excellent people in the alternative health industry, who are very experienced, have good knowledge in their area of expertise, practise safely and get great results, there seems to be an inordinate number of people working in this area who take such extreme approaches that they may be putting your health at risk. I am not saying this just from what I have heard other people say. I take a huge interest in all approaches to health and wellbeing and have taken the time to explore them myself, too – or else I wouldn't be able to comment credibly.

The number of people I have met who have been told to cut out entire food groups for months on end from a 20-minute consultation or looking at a strand of hair or the back of the tongue is unreal. I have also spoken with many people who have been advised to take an excessive number of supplements without having a thorough health examination first or without even a consideration of what they are currently eating. It is my belief that supplements have a time and a place, which is when there is a clearly defined reason to be taking them, not just swallowing them down without good reason – more isn't always better.

Also, in some cases, extreme approaches can breed beliefs about the need to 'diet', 'restrict' and follow 'rules' as well as beliefs that food can be somehow 'good' or 'bad'. I have worked with so many people who end up with a very disordered relationship with food after previously receiving unsound, unrealistic advice. So, it really pays, therefore, to be careful about who you are taking advice from. It is often far less clear to see how qualified the person is, as some areas of alternative health don't seem to be that well regulated.

There are certainly some interesting and exciting ideas which come from the alternative health camp, but you can probably now see that those with a medical background struggle with the concepts and beliefs of some alternative approaches. So there you have it – how debates, disagreements, conflicting newspaper and magazine articles are born. There are so many sides to each story!

A combined approach

A term commonly used these days is that of 'integrative' or 'complementary' medicine, which basically means that some alternative approaches are taken alongside what is considered traditional medicine. This is becoming increasingly popular and is seen as a more holistic approach by some. Watch this space, I guess – there will no doubt be some interesting developments coming up; but again, please be careful who you listen to – not everyone is really the expert they may claim to be.

CONFUSION IS BORN

You can now see that if you ask two people in the health world the same question, you are open to a number of different answers depending on who you ask, what they have learnt and what they believe to be true.

Let's take butter, for example – a massively debated topic. From the medical point of view, based on hard, sound, good-quality research, we know that saturated fat from animal origins is a huge contributor to heart disease. Butter is the second biggest source of saturated fat in the New Zealand diet and it doesn't take a rocket scientist to work out that reducing the amount of butter and replacing it with healthier fats can assist (and has been proven to assist) with reducing the rates of heart disease and so save lives.

However, the perspective of many alternative health professionals is that because butter is natural (so is arsenic by the way) it is okay for you to eat it. Now, if you are a relatively healthy individual, having the odd bit of butter here and there is okay; in truth, swapping from butter to an alternative (although I would still recommend it) might only make a small difference to your heart disease risk. But for the people who are the most at risk of getting heart disease, who eat fatty meats, deep-fried foods and large amounts of butter each day, this is a change that could save their lives.

The hype around margarines and spreads being two molecules away from plastic are simply untrue. Yes, they are manufactured products and yes, they are processed, but it doesn't mean they will kill you. If you don't like the idea of including them for your own reasons, that's fine, you don't have to. But I wouldn't suggest hitting the butter hard as an alternative; instead, try using avocado, nut butters or hummus as a spread and healthy oils in cooking – all round that makes for a win–win situation, no drama needed.

Historically there seemed to be fewer conflicting stories in the media about health and wellbeing, so a lay person would have had less trouble figuring out the messages health experts were trying to get across. Now, though, with opinions from both sides of the spectrum in magazines, newspapers, TV and radio – alongside the opinions of those who have no formal training but feel like they are an expert in the topic after following a certain diet, reading a book or just having come to their own conclusion on things – messages are getting all mixed up and there is no wonder people are so confused.

BE MINDFUL

Check your expert's qualifications

Over the years I have noticed that more and more people seem to see themselves as experts in nutrition. These days, anyone can call themselves a nutritionist, nutrition expert or nutrition consultant without any formal training or qualifications and, of course, as with any topic, everyone is entitled to their own opinion. My advice is to always check your dietitian or nutritionist's qualifications.

- Dietitians are registered health professionals who have completed a three-year undergraduate degree in human nutrition and a further one year post-graduate diploma in dietetics. They are specifically trained to work in a variety of settings and practise nutrition based on the best scientific evidence.
- Nutritionists can vary from those who have a three-year science degree in human nutrition to those who have done an online course or just choose to call themselves a nutritionist, so it is important to check who is giving you advice.

Friends or colleagues with good intentions, but no background

If you have tried something yourself and it works, what do you do? Tell people, of course! That is human nature; but the problem is, it doesn't mean it is right for everyone. Just be mindful of those who have tried a certain diet which seems to be working for them, particularly if it seems quite extreme. If you know someone who has read a book or a few things online and spread the magic words about totally overhauling the way you eat, cutting out this, that and the other, keep your eyes wide open – is this really a good long-term solution? When I say long term, I mean years, not months.

Don't get me wrong, I am all for sharing good ideas, helping people out and wanting to spread the word about eating well and getting the most from yourself but, in my experience, sometimes a little bit of knowledge can be dangerous.

Gym instructors and personal trainers

Question: If you were going to get your car washed, would you ask the guy washing your car why your engine is making a funny noise or if your suspension is safe?
Answer: Probably not.

Just because someone works with cars in some way, doesn't mean they know everything about cars or that they have the knowledge or experience to be able to advise you on all car-related matters.

The fitness industry is much the same, and I can say that with absolute confidence being a qualified fitness instructor and trainer myself, having worked in the industry and having many friends in the industry as well as training at the gym most days. There are so many mixed messages being given out by trainers – with the best intentions, I am sure – which don't really help if you end up getting yourself all confused!

There will be some trainers who are indeed qualified in nutrition (with more than a 12-week internet course, I would hope), have good experience and knowledge and will be able to offer a balanced perspective on nutrition. However, much like the car-washing example, do not assume that because someone works in the fitness industry, they have any training or a reputable background in the area of nutrition. It may be that you are given advice based on what works for that trainer or what they have read in books or online, but you still need to be mindful of information you are being given, particularly if it seems extreme, involves cutting out a vast number of foods, is very restrictive, and buckets of supplements are recommended.

The reason I say this is not because their approach won't work in the short term – it probably will – but, as I will show you throughout this book, following overly restrictive eating plans without changing your behaviours and managing triggers is only likely to lead to a dysfunctional relationship with food. Restricting food and food types can lead to binge cycles and you may end up weighing more in the long run – boy, have I seen this happen to people too many times.

Supplement sellers

Be very mindful of those with no formal qualifications in nutrition or medicine who are selling supplements; they are very unlikely to have a good understanding of the underlying physiology of the human body and are sometimes unable to see that one size doesn't fit all. I have heard many horror stories about people being sold supplements at coffee groups, dinner parties and other social gatherings by unqualified people who are making money from selling these things as part of a pyramid scheme, and who don't have a good understanding of the individual's full medical history and background.

It is all about the context . . .

When people ask me how long it takes to train to be a dietitian, they are shocked at my response that it takes four years of full-time study and training – and that is just the beginning. 'It's just food, isn't it? Can't be that tricky' is a reply I have heard a hundred times. Although, I grant you, food does seem pretty straightforward, what happens to food after you have eaten is a fascinating, complicated and an intricate, incredibly complex chain of events.

To demonstrate my point, let's side-step for just one minute and look at another example of what also at first might seem like a pretty straightforward concept – building your own deck. This is probably more a female point of view, I admit, but when you think about it, how hard can it be to build a big deck outside your property – you know, one with room for a barbecue to enjoy in summer? Surely it is just putting down some wood and knocking in some nails, right? If you have read a bit about it, tried building the odd thing here and there, surely it can't be that hard – you could do it if you had a spare weekend, right?

But when you think about it a bit more, how do you make sure the wood is all put together correctly, or that the wood doesn't break, crack or rot in the first few years? You can read all about how to do it from a book and online, but that doesn't always make it any easier when you come to start building a deck yourself. As with so many things, you don't know what you don't know, and that is where mistakes start happening. You didn't know you needed to think about some stuff until things started going wrong and you had to find a solution to fix them.

If you want a deck built, my guess is you would want to make sure that the person who puts it together understands all the possible things that could happen to it over time, and all the ways in which things could affect it or compromise its long-term durability. The person responsible for such decisions wouldn't just know how to put the wood together, but would ideally have the knowledge, skills and experience to make the process of building a deck run smoothly. They would know things you couldn't possibly know if you were new to building and outdoor renovations!

As you can see, what might seem like a straightforward concept can be more complex than you think. I often say to people who have read one article about a current food 'trend' or 'scare' that it isn't what they know about that trend or scare that is important, but rather how 'true' or relevant it is in the bigger picture of their life and health. If you believed every hype or fear around food, I bet you would be living your life on the edge of your seat thinking everyone is out to kill and poison you – how totally exhausting and unhealthy! What you lack, without a good background to how the body works and what happens when you eat and drink, is an ability to apply context and it is my belief that context is critical.

When someone tries to simplify a message about nutrition without understanding the context of the bigger picture, the outcome of the interpretation can be completely wrong and, quite frankly, add yet another level of confusion to an already complicated topic.

As you may know, I am one of the nutritionists for *Healthy Food Guide* magazine here in New Zealand and one of the things I absolutely love about that magazine is that it is one of the only sources of print media which commits to only publishing up-to-date, CREDIBLE information and its aim is to always apply context.

START WITH THE BIGGER PICTURE

Regardless of all the differing opinions and ideas out there, I actually think the most important thing when it comes to your health and reaching your goals in the first instance is to never forget the 'bigger picture'. For the most substantial effect on your overall health and wellbeing, it's really about what you eat and drink most of the time, the majority of your life. The annual 12-week challenge, stopping drinking for a month along with the odd bout of going to the gym may make a small impact on how long you live and how good you feel but, really, what makes the most significant difference is the way you live your life when it comes to food and drink — consistently eating the foods your body needs and being able to moderate and minimise the stuff it doesn't.

For me to help you get in the best shape of your life, lose weight, keep it off and feel fabulous forever, I'm looking to help you set up healthy eating habits and behaviours which last a lifetime and allow you to be consistent about the way that you eat. Really and truthfully it's what you do all the time that counts — not a year or two on supplements or a few rounds of dieting.

Just recently I was talking to a good friend about someone we both know who is currently following a very restrictive diet. Right now she is looking quite good, but all she talks about is food and what she can and can't eat. She will take pretty much any pill or potion people tell her to in the hope that it will keep her slim — but, deep down, I suspect, she isn't happy at all, even with her new slim thighs.

Food is now ruling her life and, I imagine, it will continue to do so until she is willing to take a different approach, one that she can sustain. I know changing the way you think and feel about food isn't as glam as meal replacement shakes with a picture of a skinny girl on the front, but there is a reason why the dieting industry is so massive and makes so much money, because so much of it doesn't REALLY work long term, so you have to move on to the next big thing. I feel so lucky to be doing what I do now and not getting caught up in all that rubbish. I hope by the end of this book you will be able to distance yourself from all that hype, too — it's so unhelpful.

DON'T BUY INTO OBSESSION

I firmly believe that some people today are far too obsessed with what they eat, to the point that it is unhealthy. They count every kilojoule, eliminate whole food groups at the drop of a hat, worry about everything they put in their mouths and no longer take any enjoyment from eating.

There is a term for people who have an obsession with healthy eating and it's called orthorexia. Seriously, I swear, there are some people who will drop dead as a result of their anxiety and fear of food before they will ever suffer any negative effects of poor nutrition! There is a balance between a healthy interest in eating and being obsessive – don't lose sight of that. You won't live longer just because you know the kilojoule content of foods better than the person next door, and on your death bed do you really want to be thinking 'I spent my whole life obsessing about food when I could have been living'?

Part 2: The Lose Weight for Life approach – eat for the right reasons

My approach to nutrition is a practical one and in Lose Weight for Life I have been able to combine my knowledge of dietetics with my research into all areas of nutrition practice and my experience of working with thousands of people. I want to help and encourage you to enjoy a variety of foods, to eat when you're hungry and to get the balance of nutrients you need for your body to work at its best, as well as supporting you to have a healthy relationship with the food you eat.

So, the time has finally come to clear up any misunderstandings, myths and confusion about what is best to eat by going right back to the beginning. We will look at the function of food, at what happens to your food after you have eaten, and from there build you a plan to move forwards.

THE FUNCTION OF FOOD

Food is the nourishment for every cell in your body; it provides the energy and goodness you need to think, move, walk, talk and be. Worldwide, the sharing of food unites friends and families, and allows people to display their creative side by preparing delicious culinary delights from the simplest snacks to the most decadent meals.

We eat when we are peckish, bored, because it's 12.30 which means it's lunchtime, or when food is free. We eat when people offer us new things to try, when we are happy, sad, angry, tired and sometimes just because it is there. But, I raise a question: even though food tastes nice and you enjoy eating it, why do you actually NEED to eat at all?

At first this might seem like a very straightforward (and possibly ridiculous) question, but I do have good reason to ask it. At the start of most of my workshops and seminars I always ask people why they think they need to eat and I am sometimes gobsmacked by the responses.

Here is a typical scenario:

> **Claire:** So, this might seem like a silly question, but why do we need to eat?
> **Audience:** (always someone at the back) For energy!
> **Claire:** Excellent, that is right . . . are there any other reasons why we need to eat?

Audience: Fuel?

Claire: Yes, that is also right – food is the fuel or energy we need to make our bodies work. But here are other questions for you: What do you need this energy for? What does your body do every day that needs energy?

Audience: (silence, most commonly accompanied by blank faces)

It is clear that the message that food is fuel has got through to people, but, I guess, having an understanding of what the body uses this fuel for hasn't been made clear enough. Food provides the fuel or the energy that you need to keep your body working and doing all the amazing, magical, wonderful and spectacular things it does on a daily basis that we all take for granted. Food gives you the energy you need to move your arms and legs, for your lungs to expand and contact, for your liver to take its punishment on a Friday night after a wine session. It gives you the energy your brain needs to think, process information and make decisions for you, for your eyes to blink, muscles to grow and for your kidneys to filter the 1500 litres of blood that they thanklessly do each and every day without you even asking them to.

Why your body needs food

There are so many reasons why you need to eat. Here are a few examples:

BRAIN		To supply your **brain** with the fuel it needs. Your brain uses around 20 per cent of the kJ your body needs each day. It also needs essential fats to function.
HEART		To allow your **heart** to beat and pump blood around your body.
LIVER		To allow your **liver** to metabolise the food you eat as well as process alcohol, drugs and hormones.
KIDNEYS		To enable your **kidneys** to filter your blood.
MUSCLES		To supply your **muscles** with the energy they need so that you can move around.

Did you know?
- Every hour around 1 billion cells in your body are replaced.
- Your kidneys filter around 1500 litres of blood every day.
- Your heart pumps around 35 million times a year.
- At any given time about 5 per cent of your bones are being broken down and being rebuilt.

The human body, in my mind, is just incredible, and the more you understand about how amazing it is the more it upsets you to see how much people take their bodies for granted and abuse them – and then complain about them breaking down and not working properly . . . but that's another story.

WHAT IS YOUR ROLE IN ALL THIS?

You have a choice about what you put in your mouth. You have the choice of what you buy, what you cook and what combinations of food and drink you have each day. You have the ability to control the type of fuel that you put into your body. It is your job to look after yourself the best you can, for yourself and for those around you so you can live a long, healthy, happy life. Of course, success, as you will by now be very aware of, is not just what you know, but what you do: your habits, behaviours and beliefs when it comes to food (we will come to this in more detail, I promise). But still, first up, it's vital to have some clarity on what you need to be eating and how much.

HOW MUCH DO YOU NEED TO EAT?

Essentially, the amount that people need to eat varies depending on their gender, body composition, level of activity and stage of life – this is why you can't take a one-size-fits-all approach to nutrition. I have said it before and will no doubt say it again: we are, thank heavens, all different!

Your kilojoule budget

Your body needs energy (fuel) to allow your brain to work, muscles to move and heart to beat, as I have already discussed. The amount of energy your body needs to do everything on a daily basis is measured in kilojoules or kilo-calories (calories). I call this your kilojoule budget.

Did you know?

- Kilojoules (kJ) and kilocalories (kcal) mean exactly the same thing. They are just two different units, much like centimetres and inches which both measure length, but are different units. In this book I will use kilojoules as it is the measurement most commonly used in New Zealand.
- To convert kilojoules to kilocalories, just divide by 4.
  4 kJ = 1 kcal.
- The food that you eat all contains kilojoules, but the amount varies depending on what type of food you are eating. A large carrot has 97 kJ and a giant biscuit has 2000 kJ.

There is no ideal way to work out how many kilojoules or how much energy you need, but the most common way is to use a bunch of complicated equations. These basically look at your age and weight and work out roughly how many kilojoules you need for your body to do the very basics on a day-to-day basis. The figure you get from these equations is known as your basal metabolic rate (BMR). On top of this is added an activity factor to account for how active a person is.

Based on averages, the recommendation is for New Zealand adults to have roughly 8700 kJ a day. This is the figure used to calculate percentages of energy on food labels in New Zealand, so when you see that one serving of something is 7 per cent of your daily intake (as in the nutrition information panel below), what this means is it is 7 per cent of 8700 kJ.

Nutrition information
Servings per package: 12
Average serving size: 40 g (²/₃ metric cup)

	Quantity per serving	% daily intake per serving	Per 100 g
Energy (kJ)	600 kJ	7%	1490 kJ
Protein	3.5 g	7%	8.8 g
Fat, total – Saturated	0.8 g 0.1 g	1% 0.5%	1.9 g 0.3 g
Carbohydrate – Sugars	28.3 g 6.4 g	9% 7%	70.7 g 15.9 g
Dietary fibre	3.6 g	12%	9 g

At the most simplistic level, when you eat the same number of kilojoules each day – the amount that you need to think, keep your heart beating and your body moving around – then in theory your weight will stay the same. Logically, then, if you eat more kilojoules than you need, your body can't use them, so it stores them; if you eat less than you need, the opposite happens and you lose weight. Essentially this is true, but there are so many other factors which affect your weight. As you will see later on in the section on weight-loss theory (see pages 75–81), it's not actually that straightforward.

Despite this upfront discussion on the importance of kilojoules, it is really important to say RIGHT now that counting kilojoules is not my primary focus – my approach to weight loss is helping people to optimise their nutrition. Working on dramatically increasing the frequency that you eat foods which your body needs – wholesome real foods which nourish your body – and by default cutting back on those foods which your body doesn't need is the overall goal; and, of course, eating the right amount. However, it is also helpful to get your head around the concept of kilojoules as they are a useful tool to help you compare different foods and work out what is an appropriate serving size of a given food. Throughout the book I will be giving examples of the kilojoule content of foods, comparing the kilojoules in different-sized portions of meals and snacks, and I have also included kilojoules in the recipes I've put at the back. There is no need to live with your calculator in your pocket and get too obsessed with every single kilojoule – bigger picture, remember.

Note: if you want to know exactly how many kilojoules you need per day, it is really best to see someone who can look at you, your health and your life in total. The team at Mission Nutrition can help if this is something you want to do: www.missionnutrition.co.nz.

Spending your kilojoule budget

For your body to work at its best and for you to feel like you can jump out of bed in the morning ready for a fabulous day, it REALLY matters what types of food you get your kilojoules from. You could essentially argue that if you had two cheeseburgers at around 1600 kJ each and a can of fizzy drink at 650 kJ, this is lower than your energy needs for a day, and so you would lose weight. You probably would, but it is a really unhealthy way to do it. You will be lacking vitamins, minerals and other nutritional goodness that your brain needs and that every cell in your body demands – that is not a great way to live.

For good health and wellbeing, to keep your organs working well and every part of your body in good nick, I cannot stress enough how vital it is to eat the right things and spend your kilojoule budget wisely. Let's be honest, blowing it all on cheese and crackers or bottles of wine won't get you the result you are after. Your body is simply a machine that needs looking after and you can't expect it to work wonders for you if you don't respect it.

Each day, you are looking to get the right balance of carbohydrate, protein, fat, fibre, vitamins and minerals to maximise the health and functioning of your body. If you fall short on any of these for long enough, your body won't be able to work as well as it should. Without adequate carbohydrate you can feel faint, dizzy and can lose concentration; without adequate iron (a mineral) you can look very pale, feel tired and compromise your immunity. Every food category has a place.

NUTRIENTS

Nutrients are the building blocks of all food which are made up of different combinations of carbohydrate, protein, fat, fibre, vitamins and minerals. Bread, for example, is mostly carbohydrate with some protein, fibre, a small amount of fat and a combination of various vitamins and minerals. Chicken is mostly protein, with a small amount of fat, and some vitamins and minerals.

On food labels, you will see under the nutrition information panel a column which says 'per 100 g'. Underneath this is a breakdown of the energy, protein, fat, carbohydrate, fibre, vitamins and minerals. There will be numbers next to each of these nutrients and these tell you what proportion of the 100 g of food you are buying is coming from that nutrient.

Nutrition information: cereal Serving size: 30 g Servings per package: 24			
	Per serve	Per 100 g	30 g with ½ cup (125 ml) reduced-fat milk
Energy (kJ) – (kCal)	441 105	1470 352	690 165
Protein (g)	3.6	12.0	8.1
Fat, total (g) – Saturated (g)	0.4 0.1	1.4 0.3	2.3 1.4
Carbohydrate (g) – Sugars (g)	20.1 0.8	67.0 2.8	26.1 6.8
Dietary fibre (g)	3.2	10.5	3.2

Let's look at a cereal packet (see above). When considering what this food is made of, you can see that the cereal has per 100 g: 12 g of protein, 1.4 g of fat (of which 0.3 g is saturated), 67 g of carbohydrate (of which 2.8 g is sugars – sugars are a type of carb), 10.5 g of fibre. There is also a range of different vitamins and minerals (not shown).

Why don't the numbers add up to 100 g, though, you might ask (or you may have never even noticed!)? Well, the reason is that water is not on the nutrition information panel – the number of grams of water is missing. Here, around 9 g will be water – this is the difference between 100 g and the total weights of the carbs plus protein plus fat plus fibre.

The skills of label reading are discussed later in Section Three (pages 143–6), but for now the message to take from here is that foods are made up of a mixture of different nutrients. At this point, another helpful thing to understand is that if a product is modified to be lower in a certain nutrient, then something else has to be added back in. For example, if the amount of fat in a food is reduced from 40 g per 100 g to 20 g, then 20 g of something else has to go in to replace the 20 g of fat taken out – and this may be sugar or something else.

How much of each nutrient do you need?

The amount of each of these nutrients that your body needs depends on your age and stage, your gender, how active you are and whether you have any specific health issues which may change your needs – much like your energy needs.

Here we will consider the needs of an average adult, based on someone who consumes around 8700 kJ per day. Your needs may be slightly different, but this is at least a starting point to help you get your head around the concept!

CARBOHYDRATE

What is carbohydrate?

Carbohydrate includes sugars and starches:

- **Sugars:** there are many different types of sugars; the most common types we see include sucrose (table sugar), fructose (fruit sugar) and lactose (milk sugar).
- **Starches:** these are essentially long chains of sugars joined together and come in all sorts of shapes and sizes.

Why does your body need carbohydrate?

Carbohydrate is the preferred source of fuel for the brain and muscles. The amount your body needs is hugely variable depending on your level of activity.

Your body can make carbohydrate itself from breaking down other nutrients, but for good health it is recommended that you eat foods containing carbohydrate so that your body doesn't need to do that! It is ideal to include wholegrain, starchy carbohydrate every day, as not only do these foods provide you with the fuel your brain, muscles and other body cells need, but they also provide other vital vitamins and minerals. If you are very active, you will need more carbohydrate to fuel your muscles during training and to assist with recovery.

Which foods contain carbohydrate?

- Fruits and vegetables
- Grains and cereals, including rice, pasta, couscous, bread, crackers, noodles, quinoa, oats and breakfast cereals
- Pulses such as lentils, chickpeas, kidney beans and butter beans
- Dairy products, like milk, yoghurt and ice cream
- Lollies, cakes, chocolate, biscuits, jam and honey.

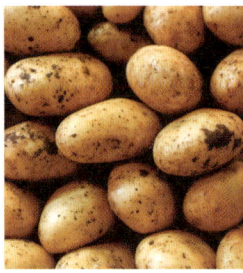 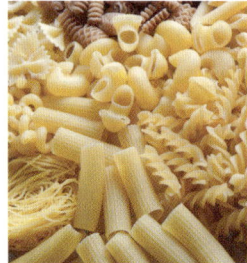 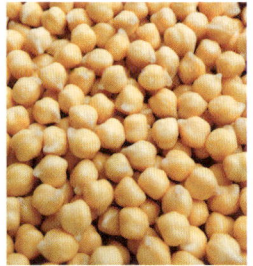

What is the glycaemic index?

The glycaemic index (GI) measures the rate at which carbohydrate-containing foods are broken down in your body. For weight management and good health, it can be helpful to base your diet on healthy carbohydrate-rich foods which have a low GI. Be mindful, though, that just because a food has a low GI, it doesn't automatically make it healthy; for example, many ice creams have a low GI, but that doesn't make them good everyday food choices. The GI is best used to compare similar foods within each food group (breads to other breads, cereals to other cereals, and so on) and it really is a tool to be used in conjunction with what you already know about smart eating.

How much carbohydrate do you need?

Carbohydrate-containing foods provide energy as well as a range of valuable vitamins and minerals and are a key part of a healthy balanced diet – but the HOW MUCH question is really important to consider.

The Ministry of Health recommends we get 45–65 per cent of our energy from carbohydrate-containing foods. Based on the average of 8700 kJ a day, this works out to around 235–340 g per day. This figure includes both starches and sugars, but for good health we would like the sugar component to be as low as possible – particularly the added sugars. We are looking for the majority to come from whole grains, fruits, vegetables and legumes, rather than processed starches and sugars.

If your goal is to lose weight, you are likely to be consuming less than 8700 kJ per day; a sensible starting point for a moderately active adult would be around 6000 kJ per day. The exact amount will need to be calculated for you individually based on your current weight, age and level of activity, so please be mindful that this figure of 6000 kJ is just to be used as an example, rather than a personalised prescription.

When you aim to lose weight and have a lower intake of kilojoules each day, the amount of carbohydrate you will need will also be less. As we are all different, it is impossible to give a definitive number of grams to aim for each day without speaking to you first, so rather than getting out the calculator, let's focus on the practical things you can do when it comes to eating the right amount for you:

- Look to include 2 servings of fruit and 3 + handfuls of non-starchy vegetables (especially greens!) each and every day. You don't need more fruit than this if you are watching your waistline; best to stock up on the lower-carb veggies than have too much fruit sugar.
- When you are having breakfast cereal, porridge or bircher muesli, you don't need a massive huge bowlful! Stick to $\frac{1}{2}$–1 cup max in most cases (of course, this will depend on what it is).
- With your grains and other starchy foods, as well as ALWAYS going for the wholegrain option when you can, don't cook more than you need: $\frac{1}{2}$–1 cup cooked grains or starchy food per serving is likely to be adequate for a meal. The same applies to your starchy veggies such as potatoes, kumara, yams, taro and green bananas.

- If you are making a soup, casserole, curry or tasty dish which is packed with lentils, chickpeas or any other type of legume, remember these are high in carbohydrate and you are unlikely to need extra bread, rice or pasta with it – and if you do, don't overdo it!
- Have as little carbohydrate in the form of sugar as is possible. Start reducing the amount of sugar you add to things until you get used to having none at all, if possible. Swap to unsweetened yoghurt – you will get used to it. Keep well clear of sugary drinks too – you just don't need them.

PROTEIN

What is protein?

Protein is a combination of smaller building blocks known as amino acids. There are 22 different types of amino acids in total, like 22 different coloured marbles. These amino acids are found in food and are joined together in different combinations. In meat, poultry, fish and eggs you will find all 22 of the amino acids and, therefore, these foods are known as complete protein foods. Baked beans, nuts, seeds and other plant proteins only have some of these 22 amino acids in them and are known as incomplete protein foods.

Why does your body need protein?

Despite the fact that your body may look pretty much the same tomorrow as it does today, it will be slightly different. Your body is constantly being broken down and rebuilt in a slow and steady process. You lose hair which needs replacing, red blood cells die and new ones are needed, and your bones are constantly being remade. This rebuilding process, as well as everyday wear and tear on the body, requires protein. Different amino acids are needed for different jobs, and for good overall health and wellbeing you need a whole variety of these so that all your body's jobs can get done properly.

Which foods contain protein?

- Meat, poultry, seafood (such as fish, prawns, mussels, oysters) and eggs
- Milk, yoghurt and cheese
- Nuts and seeds
- Pulses
- Tofu
- Grains and cereals.

How much protein do you need?

The Ministry of Health's recommendation is that 15–25 per cent of our total energy per day comes from protein (that's from the total number of kilojoules

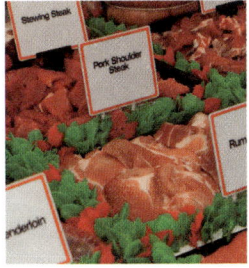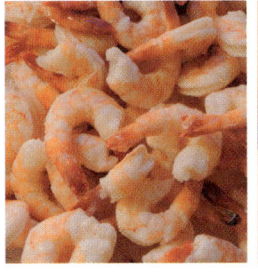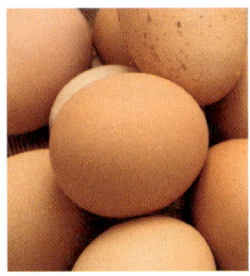

you need in a day). Based on the average intake of 8700 kJ a day, this is around 78–130 g of protein per day. Another way protein requirements are calculated is based on the number of grams your body needs per kilogram of your body weight. This will need to be individually calculated. Those of you who are very active and do a significant amount of resistance training may need more protein than those who are more sedentary.

My recommendation when it comes to protein is to try to include protein-rich foods in each of your meals. Aim to spread your protein throughout the day, rather than doing what most people tend to do which is having very little at breakfast and lunch and a massive dose at night with a big steak or something similar for dinner – this isn't helpful for your body.

The most recent findings suggest that the majority of people in New Zealand have an adequate amount of protein in their diet. It is perfectly possible to get all the protein you need from everyday foods. With a few serves of dairy and meat or fish in a day, most people can very easily meet their needs for protein. For vegetarians, it just takes a little more time to make sure you get enough from alternative sources to meat and fish.

Here's the protein content of some common foods:

- 1 size 7 egg = 6 g
- 150 g lean steak (raw weight) = 35 g
- 150 g skinless chicken (raw weight) = 33 g
- 150 g white fish (raw weight) = 30 g
- 100 g can tuna = 26 g
- 150 g tofu = 12 g
- 1 pottle low-fat yoghurt = 7 g
- 1 cup trim milk = 11 g
- 1 cup kidney beans = 15 g
- 1 cup baked beans = 11 g.

(Data gathered from Foodworks 2009)

Why are some people obsessed with protein?

There has been huge interest in and a tremendous amount of research on the area of high-protein, low-carbohydrate diets, and the trend still seems highly popular today. While protein has some hugely important roles in the body, is high on the satiety ratings and is believed to be helpful in supporting weight loss, there is a misconception that more is always better. There is no need to eat whole chickens, endless cans of tuna and protein shakes galore to achieve a healthy weight and a lean body. Having more than 2 g protein per kilogram of your body weight has been shown to have no additional benefits. To put that into perspective, a 70 kg person eating 2 g of protein per kilogram of body weight equals 140 g of protein per day.

The pro-protein message often goes hand in hand with a degree of carb phobia and, I know, for many people can mean serious restriction of their carbohydrate intake, which is neither necessary or healthy. It is fine to make sure that you are getting the protein you need (remember, most of us are already), but it is not necessary to combine this with carbohydrate restriction – there is absolutely nothing wrong with including an APPROPRIATE amount of healthy whole grains, fruits, vegetables and legumes in your daily eating as well.

Protein bars and shakes

There is a time and a place for protein bars, drinks and powders. They can be quick, convenient and helpful after training for those who are doing very regular, high-intensity exercise or resistance training. However, please don't think that taken independently these products will help you get the body of your dreams. They are often heavily processed, packed with sweeteners and flavourings, and very expensive. The combination of eating healthy balanced meals and snacks and doing the right exercise programme for you is what will get you the results you want. There are also some protein shakes and bars that are very high in kilojoules and have far more in a serving than you would actually need. If you are taking these, be sure you are using them for the right reasons.

FAT

What is fat?

Fat comes in different shapes and sizes and is sometimes referred to as the good and bad or healthy and unhealthy fat. Fat often gets a bad rap, but there is no doubt at all that including some fat in your diet is very important, not to mention incredibly good for you! Foods containing fat also carry the fat-soluble vitamins A, D, E and K which are vital for health and wellbeing. When it comes to fat, the trick is making sure you are getting them from the right places – more of the fat with healthy benefits and less of those which are not helpful for your body.

Saturated fat and trans-fat

These types of fat are often known as the ones that encourage your body to make the bad type of cholesterol (LDL) which sticks to the inside of your blood vessels, clogging them up, which can cause heart disease.

Foods with a significant amount of saturated fat include the white fat on meat and chicken skin, and the fat in dairy foods such as cream, full-fat milk, cheese and butter. Coconut oil and coconut cream are also high in saturated fat.

There is currently some debate as to whether all types of saturated fat have the same effect on your body and there is work being done to see if there are some which are more detrimental than others. But more research is needed; so, I guess, as with all science . . . we will see what comes up.

Be mindful of trans-fat – you really want to avoid this at all costs. Pastries, cakes and biscuits are likely to be the worst offenders here.

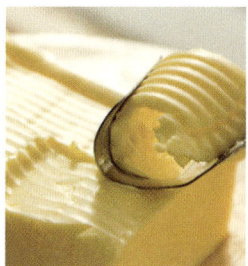 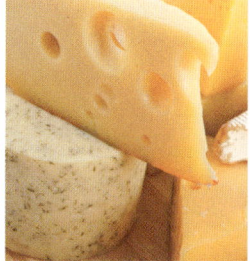 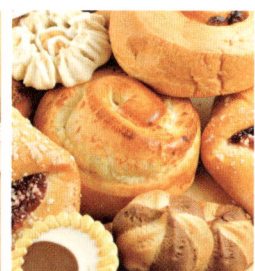

Unsaturated fat

Unsaturated fat is categorised by its chemical structure and is either mono-unsaturated or polyunsaturated. These unsaturated fats have a positive impact on health and are really important to include in your diet. Examples of foods that are high in healthy fat include nuts, seeds, oily fish, avocado, and oils or spreads made from olive, canola or ricebran.

There are certain types of polyunsaturated fats – called omega 3, 6 and 9 – which are of particular interest when it comes to good health and wellbeing. While all the omega fats are important, the ratio between them is something worth considering and in New Zealand we are currently having more of the omega 6 fat than we need relative to the amount of omega 3 fat. So, what does this mean? Well, let's get eating more fresh salmon and using oils which are higher in omega 3 and lower in omega 6. A good-quality olive oil is a great choice.

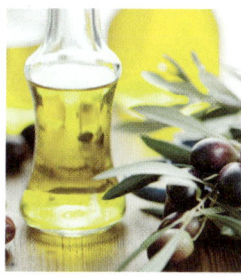 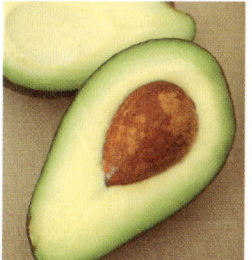 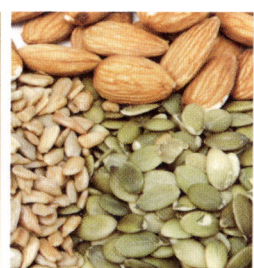

How much fat do you need?

It is recommended that we get 20–35 per cent of our daily kilojoule needs from fat; with an average intake of 8700 kJ per day, this works out to 45–80 g of fat per day. Ideally, none of this would come from trans-fat and an absolute maximum of 23 g would come from saturated fat, with the least amount possible being the goal. In New Zealand the current issue is that people are consuming far too much saturated fat and not enough of the healthy fat. For those on the waistline watch, with a base of 6000 kilojoules per day, sticking to the lower end of this fat range is preferable, with as much of the fat as possible coming from healthy foods!

FIBRE

What is fibre?

Fibre is the indigestible portion of plant foods. There are lots of different ways to describe fibre, but one of the simplest is to consider fibre in these terms:

> **Soluble fibre:** this type of fibre acts like a sponge, absorbing fluid and making the contents of the bowel softer and allowing things to move through more easily.
> **Insoluble fibre:** acts as a bulking agent and works with the soluble fibre to help things move through your digestive system more easily.

Why does your body need fibre?

Fibre helps things move through your digestive system, keeps you 'regular' and helps you to feel full. Having plenty of fibre can also help to reduce the risk of heart disease, some cancers and diabetes.

Which foods contain a significant amount of soluble fibre?

- Oats
- Legumes, such as dried peas, beans and lentils
- Vegetables, especially broccoli, Brussels sprouts, carrots, potatoes and kumara
- Fruit, especially apples, pears, citrus, stonefruit and berryfruit.

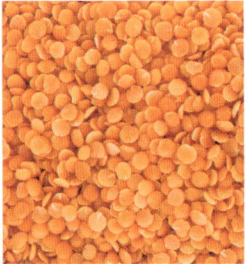 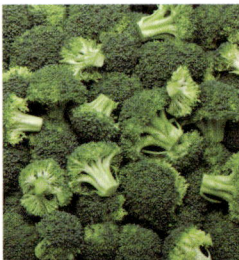 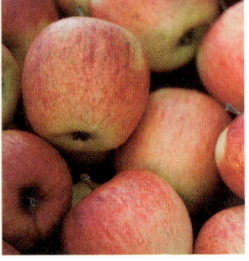

Which foods contain a significant amount of insoluble fibre?

- Breads, such as mixed grain, wholemeal
- Wholegrain cereals
- Whole-wheat pasta
- Brown rice
- Corn and cornmeal or polenta
- Fruits and vegetables.

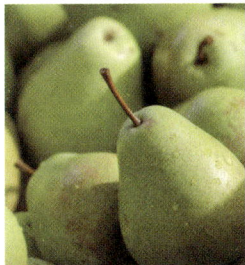 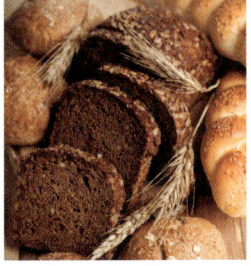 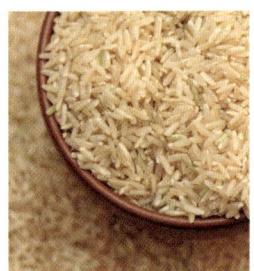

Along with both well-known types of fibre, there is something called resistant starch which acts rather like a third type of fibre. It doesn't get digested as it passes through the gut, but when it hits the large intestine (colon) it is used as a food source for bacteria; this is a great thing as, during this process, some really helpful compounds are produced which keep the bowel in good working order.

There is a lot of interesting research coming through about resistant starch and in time it may become clear that it actually plays a huge role in our health and wellbeing – even more so than the well-known soluble fibre and insoluble fibre.

But where do you get it from? Pulses are a great source, so get onto your chickpeas and lentils. Cooked and cooled pearl barley, brown rice, whole-wheat pasta, potatoes and unripe bananas are good, too.

How much fibre do you need?

The recommendation is for women to have at least 25 g of fibre per day and for men to have at least 30 g per day, regardless of whether you are trying to lose weight or not. This includes both soluble fibre and insoluble fibre. The bad news is that most Kiwis aren't getting enough of these types of fibre at all, with women on average eating a mere 17.5 g per day and men 22.1 g. There is work to be done, that is for sure!

To help make some sense of this, here is the amount of fibre in some common foods:

- 1 cup frozen mixed vegetables = 8.6 g
- ½ cup baked beans = 8.2 g
- 1 medium bran muffin = 6.3 g

- ½ cup natural muesli = 5.7 g
- 2 Weet-Bix = 5 g
- ½ cup stewed apricots = 3.8 g
- 1 cup cooked brown rice = 3.7 g
- 1 medium kumara (skin on) = 3.3 g
- 1 handful dried apricots (10 halves) = 2.7 g
- 1 cup porridge = 2.1 g
- 1 apple or banana = 2 g
- 1 slice wholegrain bread (e.g. Vogels) = 1.8 g
- 1 slice wholemeal bread = 1.6 g
- 1 slice white high-fibre bread = 1.1 g
- 1 slice white bread = 0.7 g.

(Data gathered from Foodworks 2009)

When it comes to resistant starch, the recommendations here in New Zealand are currently very unclear. In Australia, however, it is now being recommended that people aim to include 20 g of resistant starch each day for good health and wellbeing. For more information about resistant starch, visit www.csiro.com.au.

On your weight-loss journey, moving you towards better health and wellness, focusing on soluble fibre and insoluble fibre as well as resistant starch is going to be really important. Have a look at what you eat on an average day right now – are you getting enough?

Another thing to mention, while we are talking fibre, is that if you are planning to up your fibre, do it slowly over a few days or weeks rather than going mad overnight – or your guts won't thank you for it. Also, if you are increasing your fibre, you need to up your fluids, too – more water, people, you need to keep things moving!

Here are some tips to make sure you get your daily BOOST of fibre and resistant starch:

- Try wholegrain oats for breakfast; go for the big chunky ones.
- If you eat bread, go for dense wholegrain varieties.
- Choose brown rice where you can. If you soak it in the morning, it will make cooking it much quicker in the evening.
- Be sure to get your 5 + a day of fruits and veggies.
- Leave the skin on your potatoes and kumara, and other veggies where you can.
- Add a tablespoon of oat bran, wheat bran or some ground LSA (linseed, sunflower seed and almond mix) to your breakfast or to a smoothie – it will thicken it up, and tastes delicious.
- Use more pulses – make soups with lentils, add chickpeas to currries, add more kidney beans to chilli; the ideas are endless (check out the recipe section from page 216 onwards for some ideas).
- Make cold rice or pasta salads with plenty of veggies and lean meat or fish or eggs.

VITAMINS

What are vitamins?

Vitamins, although very tiny in size, are a hugely important part of the food that we eat. There are a number of different vitamins including A, B (a group of several vitamins), C, D, E and K. Vitamins play a very significant role in keeping the body working at its best. If you have an inadequate amount of any of these, your health may be compromised in both the short and the long term, and I don't need to tell you it is best to avoid this.

Here in New Zealand there are certain vitamins that people are short on. In particular, I see people who are very low in B vitamins and there are certain people who are also deficient in vitamin D. The ideal situation is for us to work on improving the quality of our diets and eating a better balance of foods to allow us to get the vitamins we need, without heading for a pot of pills as the answer. Eating good-quality, fresh, whole foods is a really great starting point and, as you will see from the following table, so is having lots and lots of green leafy veggies!

As well as making sure you are getting enough of these vitamins from your diet, it is critical to consider how well your body is able to absorb these goodies when they are inside you. Keeping your gut healthy is paramount to allowing your body to absorb the nutrients you are putting into it! More on this on page 87.

Vitamin	What is it and what do we need it for?	Where is it found?
A	Vitamin A is a fat-soluble vitamin found in two forms: 1) Retinol (in animal foods) 2) Carotenoids (in plant foods) – the most common type being beta carotene. Vitamin A is needed to help to keep your skin and eyes healthy, to improve vision at night and in dim light, and acts as an antioxidant. BEWARE: Too much vitamin A can be toxic, and can be a particular issue during pregnancy as an excess of vitamin A can lead to birth defects. Avoid eating too much liver during pregnancy or taking supplements with vitamin A in them. Seek advice if you're pregnant.	Retinol is found in liver, oily fish, and full-fat dairy products. Carotenoids are found in dark green vegetables such as silver beet, spinach and broccoli, as well as in yellow and orange vegetables such as capsicums and carrots.

Table continues overleaf

Vitamin	What is it and what do we need it for?	Where is it found?
B and folic acid (or folate)	There are a number of B vitamins, including vitamin: • B1 (thiamin) • B2 (riboflavin) • B3 (niacin) • B6 (pyridoxine) • B12 (cyanocobalamin). The B vitamins are known as water-soluble vitamins. For good health it is important to eat foods packed with B vitamins each and every day to make sure you are getting all that you need. The B vitamins help convert carbohydrate, protein and fat into energy. Vitamin B12 is needed for the body to make red blood cells as well as nerves, so is very important. Folic acid is grouped with the B vitamins and is also important in helping the body to make red blood cells. It also plays a vital role in preventing neural tube defects such as spina bifida in unborn babies.	Vitamin B1 is found in whole grains, meat, nuts and some fortified breakfast cereals. Vitamin B2 is found in milk, eggs, liver, green veggies and some fortified breakfast cereals. Vitamin B3 is found in meat and some fortified breakfast cereals. Vitamin B6 is found in beef, fish, poultry, eggs, whole grains and some vegetables. Vitamin B12 is found in meat, milk, eggs and some yeast extracts. (Vegetarians and vegans often fall short on this vitamin so may need to take supplements.) Folate is found in dark green leafy vegetables, liver, legumes, bananas, oranges, some fortified breakfast cereals and some breads.
C	Vitamin C is another water-soluble vitamin, also known as ascorbic acid. It has several important roles, including acting as an antioxidant, assisting with immunity, improving the absorption of non-haem (plant-based) iron and helping the body to make collagen which is an essential component of the skin, blood vessels, bone and teeth.	Fruits and vegetables are packed with vitamin C. On the fruit front, kiwifruit, citrus fruits and berries are the best sources. With vegetables, capsicum, tomato and green vegetables are really good sources.

Vitamin	What is it and what do we need it for?	Where is it found?
D	Vitamin D is a fat-soluble vitamin which helps to keep bones and teeth strong and healthy. The best way to get vitamin D is to help your body to make it by itself. How? By exposing your skin to sunlight – that doesn't mean frying yourself in the sun, but it means going outside and exposing at least your hands and your face to sunlight each day. Try to avoid going outside at risk times (between 10 a.m. and 3 p.m. from September through to April). Some groups of people in New Zealand are short on vitamin D – generally those who stay indoors a lot or who cover up for cultural reasons. If this sounds like you, head to your GP to talk things through.	Vitamin D is found in oily fish, eggs, lean meat and dairy products, and some fortified spreads, milks and yoghurts. Sunlight is the best way to get your vitamin D dose.
E	Vitamin E is another fat-soluble vitamin which helps to keep cell membranes healthy at the same time as acting as an antioxidant.	Vitamin E is found in nuts, seeds, avocados, spreads, vegetable oils and wheat germ.
K	Vitamin K is yet another fat-soluble vitamin which is essential to help your blood clot, and its importance should not be underestimated. Bacteria in your gut make most of the vitamin K that your body needs, but some foods contain it, too.	Vitamin K is found in green leafy vegetables, vegetable oils and some fortified milk products.

MINERALS

What are minerals?

Like vitamins, minerals are small but vital parts of the food that we eat. There is a huge number of minerals we could discuss, but the ones of most significance here in New Zealand are calcium, zinc, iodine, selenium and iron, given that these are the main ones which people appear to be falling short of. Results from the 2008/09 New Zealand National Nutrition Survey, conducted by the Ministry of Health, indicate that:

- Most people over 15 years of age aren't getting enough calcium.
- One in four adults isn't getting enough zinc, with men the bigger problem group with nearly 40 per cent not getting what they need.
- A third of men and half of women aren't getting enough selenium.
- Most people in New Zealand are mildly iodine-deficient.
- Over 7 per cent of females over the age of 15 are iron-deficient.

The good news is that if you are aware of the deficiencies that you might face, you can do something about them and prevent any negative health effects.

The next table shows which foods are good sources of each of these minerals.

Mineral	What is it and what do we need it for?	Where is it found?
Calcium	Calcium is vital to help form strong, healthy bones. It is also needed to help with muscle contracting, assist nerve function and plays a role in blood clotting.	Calcium is found in dairy products (milk, yoghurt, cheese and ice cream), fortified soy products, tofu, sardines, almonds, sesame seeds, broccoli and some fortified breakfast cereals.
Zinc	Zinc is necessary to help keep the immune system strong. It is also important to promote growth, wound healing and is vital to make healthy sperm.	Zinc is found in seafood (notably oysters and mussels), lean red meat, chicken, wholegrain cereals, legumes, seeds and dairy products.
Iron	Iron transports oxygen around the body via red blood cells. It is also an important part of many enzymes and muscle protein. There are two types of iron: • **Haem iron** is found in animal foods and is very well absorbed by the body.	Haem-iron is found in lean red meat, fish, chicken and seafood.

Mineral	What is it and what do we need it for?	Where is it found?
Iron *continued*	• **Non-haem iron** is found in plant foods and is far less well absorbed by the body. To enhance its absorption, it is best to have food or a drink rich in vitamin C at the same time.	Non-haem iron is found in wholegrain breads and cereals, eggs, vegetables, nuts, seeds and pulses.
Iodine	Iodine is necessary for thyroid function and is needed for normal growth.	Iodine is found in seafood, seaweed, eggs, dairy products, iodised salt and bread (most bread in New Zealand is now made with iodised salt).
Selenium	Selenium is a fantastic anti-oxidant, helping to keep the immune system healthy, and is also necessary for adequate thyroid function.	Selenium is found in Brazil nuts (these are the best source – adults only need 2–3 a day), eggs, fish, lean meat and grains.

So now you know what to eat and how much you need to stay healthy and well. In the following section, we will look more closely at what you need to do to lose weight.

Part 3: Weight-loss theory

There are many theories about how to lose weight and it can be a mine field trying to work out what to do! The Lose Weight for Life approach will help you understand how much to eat, ensure you are eating the right balance of foods to help your body work at its best and, very importantly, make sure that you are eating (and drinking) for all the right reasons, not because you are bored or feeling emotional. Here we will look at how much you need to eat to lose weight, plateaus, age, metabolism, and why dieting doesn't work.

FIRST, WHAT IS WEIGHT?

Let's get clear on what WEIGHT actually means in relation to the human body. The amount you weigh when you stand on the scales (be it in kilograms or stones and pounds) is the sum total of the weight of your bones, blood, organs (your brain, heart, liver and so on), muscle and fat, as well as a whole host of other small but significant things such as the bacteria that live in your gut (there is around a kilogram of them!), your nerves and much much more.

Solely judging your progress on your journey to get healthy by the number on the scales is ludicrous in my view and can be very unhelpful. This is why I asked you to look beyond mere weight when you were setting your goals. As I have previously mentioned, your weight varies at different times of the day, whether you have been to the loo or not, what time of the month it is, among other things, so please don't get too hung up on the number on the scales. You are far better to see how waist and hip measurements change over time, notice how your clothes are fitting better and that you can get into your favourite jeans again. Skin folds are also quite good if you can find someone qualified and experienced to do them for you. My advice to you if you do weigh yourself is don't do it more than once a week, and set your weight-loss goals not just on a number but on how you would like to look and feel.

LOSING WEIGHT

Taking it right to the very basics – to lose weight, or more specifically to lose body fat, you need to have less energy in the foods and drinks you consume than you are burning by being alive and moving around. A kilogram of body fat is equivalent to around several thousand kilojoules of stored fuel (somewhere around 30,000 kJ, depending on where you read about it!). But overall, by eating less than you need, you are trying to encourage your body to use some of the energy it has stored. Although starvation or eating very little may at this point seem like the most logical way to lose weight, remember that your body is cleverer than you think!

When you cut back too quickly you may indeed lose fat, but you are also at risk of losing muscle at the same time – so, yes, the number on the scales may go down, but not entirely for the right reasons. Given that muscle is the most metabolically active tissue in your body, i.e. it burns lots of kilojoules for you, the LAST thing in the world you want to be doing is burning it up. Those quick-fix options you see out there are just that, A QUICK FIX, and can breed more fat.

Your metabolic rate (the number of kilojoules your body burns per day) is also likely to drop as your body has switched to survival mode and wants to conserve its reserves rather than get rid of them – in the long term, you are doing yourself no favours. When you do eat normally again, have a binge day or decide you can no longer be on a diet, you are likely to regain weight . . . fast. And the sad thing is that you are very likely to regain fat on fat!

We all know the basics of weight loss: eat less, move more . . . But I have seen, spoken to and worked with enough people in my time to realise that this is not the whole story. There are a huge number of factors which can affect your weight and your success in losing it. The diagram opposite illustrates some of the main factors which affect your ability to lose weight and all of them need to be considered to help you get the results you want – fat which comes off and stays off. Some things you can't change (like your age, sadly), but pretty much everything else, you can – hurray!

THINGS WHICH CAN AFFECT YOUR WEIGHT AND ABILITY TO LOSE BODY FAT . . .

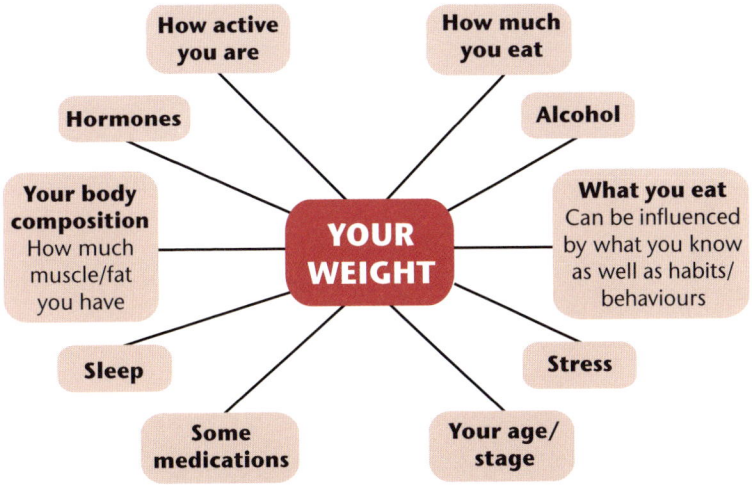

HOW MANY KILOJOULES SHOULD YOU REALLY BE EATING TO LOSE WEIGHT (WELL . . . BODY FAT)?

If you have a look online or in magazines, you will see a range of different suggestions for how many kilojoules you need to eat to lose weight. There are some endorsed by celebrities which are a mere 2000 kJ a day, to those which suggest around 4000 kJ a day, to those which are slightly more realistic at about 6000 kJ per day.

A healthy level of weight loss is around 0.5 kg a week. You need to know right here, right now that fat is a stubborn thing to shift and if you are losing weight much more quickly than that, I can pretty much guarantee initially it will be loss of water and after that it will be a combination of fat and muscle which, as I have mentioned, is UNHELPFUL. Rapid weight loss will not be all fat loss. Sorry, feel free to reach for the tissue box – the truth can hurt a little.

So we are looking for a deficit of between 2000 and 4000 kJ a day (depending on what your BMR and other needs are right now). It is important that the number you end up with isn't less than your BMR (see pages 58–9 for more on this). The only occasion when this may be recommended is before gastric surgery, when someone needs to lose a large amount of weight before being able to undergo the surgery to reduce the size of their stomach.

Stomach surgery aside, for weight loss a good place to start would be at around 6000 kJ per day (very active individuals and men are likely to need a few more kilojoules). See pages 135–8 for some 6000 kJ meal plans to help you work out how much food this actually is. But PLEASE be mindful that the exact number of kilojoules you will need is super individualised and you may need slightly less or more – this is just a ballpark to get you started. I've said it before: kilojoule counting is NOT the focus of this book, just a useful tool to help along the way. Be mindful that it is your habits and behaviours which are at the forefront of getting results here.

> **Remember:** weight loss isn't entirely logical – people lose weight at different speeds. If you are eating less than you were before and the weight is not shifting, there may be other things to consider such as your stress levels, exercise, sleep and hormones . . .

Meet Sally

Sally has just turned 50. She has spent her whole working life pushing herself to the bone at the office and has built a very successful career. With her intensely busy lifestyle, along with her love of wine, which she uses to unwind after work, getting the balance right when it comes to her nutrition has always been a low priority. She also eats when she is stressed, even though she is not hungry – normally lollies and chocolate. Now, with two teenage kids, she has unwanted extra kilos on board and really wants to get her health and wellbeing back on track for herself and her family.

Sally's weight = 78 kg   Sally's height = 1.5 m

Working with Sally, these are the things which need sorting out:

1. Energy reduction
To stay the same weight, Sally would need the New Zealand adult average of 8700 kJ per day.

To reduce her weight, I would look at lowering her intake by 2000–3000 kJ per day, so she would be looking at around 6000 kJ.

2. Dividing the kilojoule budget between meals
To help Sally work out how much to eat at each meal, I have roughly broken down her kilojoule budget into meals and snacks. This is how it worked out:

3 meals at 1600 kJ each	2 snacks at 400 kJ each	Extra (can be used to make one meal slightly bigger)	TOTAL (per day)
4800 kJ	800 kJ	400 kJ	6000 kJ

3. Getting the other things right
Remember, though, getting the kilojoules right is only one of the things we need to address to help Sally manage her weight. I would also look at:

- Improving the quality and balance of the food she eats.
- Managing stress levels.
- Establishing if there are any underlying hormonal imbalances.
- Ensuring she is getting enough good-quality sleep.
- Exercising to optimise body composition and increase muscle mass to increase metabolic rate.
- Finding an alternative to wine as a de-stresser.
- Finding an alternative to chocolate and lollies to cope with stress and pressure.

With anyone who is trying to lose weight and get healthy, the logical place to focus your attention is on kilojoule restriction or some diet plan that limits your options of food and, as a secondary result, you lose weight. But as you can see, with Sally, as with most of us, there are so many things that affect what you eat and your weight, far more than what we KNOW we should be eating. For Sally, these are time pressures, using wine to de-stress and relying on chocolate for comfort. To be successful on her health and wellness mission, the Lose Weight for Life approach is the way to go, addressing all these things! Sally can then get the long-term results she really wants.

WHY DO PEOPLE REACH PLATEAUS?

When I speak with people who are on a mission to lose weight and feel great, probably the most frustrating thing is when they feel they are doing everything they should be doing but have stopped losing weight. This often leads to people wanting to give up, losing faith and thinking that they might as well just have enjoyed wine all last week as not having it hasn't done them any favours!

Please be assured, though, this is normal and, irritatingly, more normal for some people than others. Despite the fact that part of the weight-loss puzzle is the energy-in/energy-out thing, as I have indicated above, there are SO many factors that affect your weight. Here are some of the things which might be going on:

1. When you have lost weight, say 5 kg, your body now needs slightly fewer kilojoules to maintain your body mass as there is less of you. You may need to have your BMR recalculated and, as such, it might be that to continue to lose weight you need to burn 100 or so kilojoules more or eat 100 less a day.
2. If you do the same exercise for weeks and months on end, your body will adapt and you will stop getting results. If you reach a plateau, it's time to up the intensity of your training, mix things up, add some intervals, try boxing. If you regularly run a particular route, try adding some hills or steps or running the route the opposite way.
3. Weight loss isn't LOGICAL sometimes – people are individual. Sometimes the first few kilos come off fast, then weight loss slows

down, then you may lose a few more kilos. It's important that you don't give up.

4. Your mind. In my experience, people who are highly strung, get stressed easily, like and need to be in control, want to know every kilojoule going in and out, always seem to be the ones who get to this plateau point early on. You have to believe it to do it and being mad at yourself doesn't help; neither do those stress hormones.

IT'S NOT ME, IT'S MY METABOLISM

Without any doubt, one of the most common misconceptions of people carrying more weight than they want to is that it has something to do with their metabolism being slower than someone who weighs less. Sadly, in most cases, this simply isn't true. There may be MANY things playing a part in your carrying more weight than you need to – but the slow metabolism thing is hardly ever to blame.

People who carry extra weight will actually have a higher metabolic rate than those who are smaller. This is simply because the bigger you are, the more energy is required to carry your weight. When you weigh more, your body has to work harder with every movement you make.

There is a small percentage of people who will indeed have some genuine medical issue that affects their metabolic rate, such as thyroid disorders, and there are some medications which can have an impact on the way your body uses fuel, stores body fat or which can affect appetite. This includes steroids, insulin and various drugs for psychological health issues, but for most other people it is a case of looking at the real reasons for why you are overweight.

If you really do want to boost your metabolism and burn calories more efficiently each and every day, building up your lean muscle mass is the answer. This is best done by incorporating resistance or strength training into your exercise routine several times a week and making sure you eat well after exercise to help your muscles to repair and recover.

WHY IS IT HARDER TO LOSE WEIGHT WHEN YOU GET OLDER?

It hardly seems fair: you eat well, the same as you always did, but as you get older you get fatter! This is just part of the ageing process; your body composition changes as you age and your fat mass increases and muscle mass decreases – unless you do something to change it. So, if you do exactly the same amount of exercise and eat the same at 50 as you did at 40, the like-lihood is that you will weigh more. But it is not time to give up and give in; you just require a fresh approach.

What you need to do at this point is up the exercise a bit – take your walks from 20 minutes to 30, your bike rides from 45 minutes to an hour and be sure to include resistance exercise to keep your muscle mass up. On top of this, as you get older, be mindful that you need very slightly less food each year, so consider having a tablespoon less rice at dinner, going for thinly sliced bread rather than thick, and spreading your peanut butter more sparingly. Then you will not be on a 'diet', rather you will be just very slightly tweaking things throughout your day. Also, don't get caught in the trap that good-quality or healthy foods don't affect your weight. Take oil, for example; even if you buy the best-quality olive oil on the market, it is still 480 kJ a tablespoon and that is more than a slice of bread. It is best not to be too heavy-handed.

WHY DIETING DOESN'T WORK

Every day (including the day I am writing this), I will get a call from someone telling me that they have found a magic diet that really works.

> 'I am on this diet that cuts out alcohol and sugar and I have already lost 4 kg – amazing!'
> 'I am not having carbs and protein at the same meal and it seems to be working for me – I have lost heaps of weight.'

The reason why any diet will work is because you are given a set of rules and guidelines, lists of things you can and can't eat, and the outcome is that by following this 'diet':

- You end up eating less kilojoules overall because you have to say no to things
- You end up being more focused and aware of the food you put in your mouth because you have to be in order to follow the RULES you have been set.

Therefore, the diet which tells you what to eat based on your blood type doesn't work because of some magical internal interaction caused by different foods, but because a list of instructions limits your food intake. The same goes for the cabbage soup diet, lemon detox diet, food-combining diet . . . the list goes on.

I am not suggesting that they don't deliver results in the short term, but how many people do you honestly know who have ended up healthier in the long run by doing these things? Again, I am talking years, not weeks. Not many, I bet. To get results that last, you need to set up lifelong habits and behaviours to help you to eat well – regardless of the time of day or situation.

Part 4: What happens to your food after eating?

It is one thing to spend time learning about what food should go into your mouth, but it is equally important (and I think even more fascinating!) to look at what happens to food once you have eaten it. After you've put food in your mouth, there are hundreds of thousands of things which happen to allow your body to use it for fuel, get the goodness from it and pass it to different parts of the body.

THE DIGESTIVE SYSTEM – FROM THE MOUTH TO THE BUM!

From your mouth to your bum, you basically have one long tube – a bit like a hose pipe – called the gastrointestinal (GI) tract. This has lots of different sections and each part of the tube does something different and magical, from breaking down food into tiny parts which your body can absorb and use, to getting rid of the unwanted parts of food that your body can't use, which is the 'waste' part, or poo, which comes out the other end.

We eat foods such as cereal, rice, bananas, yoghurt and cheese but the cells in your brain, kidneys and all over your body can't use food like this. Your body needs to break these foods down into their building blocks so they can be used. That means breaking the carbohydrate down into sugars, the protein into amino acids and the fat into fatty acids and glycerol. The vitamins and minerals also get separated and put to use in your body. Digestion is like putting food into a blender to break it down and then through a big sieve which separates the different components – first the food is mashed up and then divided into smaller, different parts.

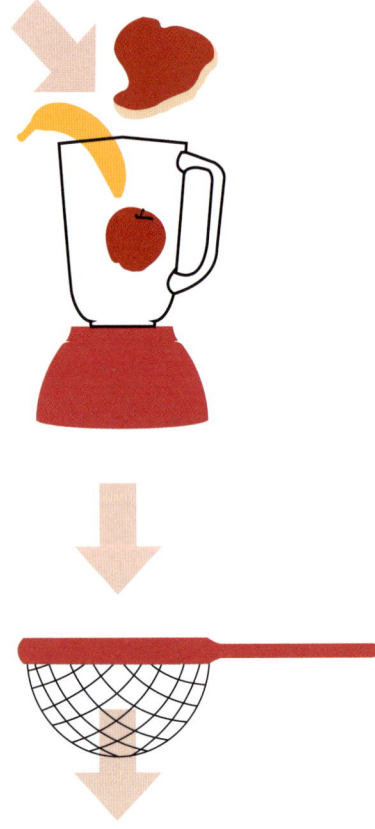

Here is a picture of the digestive system (or the magic tube!), which is a collection of organs that help break down your food. This shows you where it starts and finishes as well as where it goes on the way:

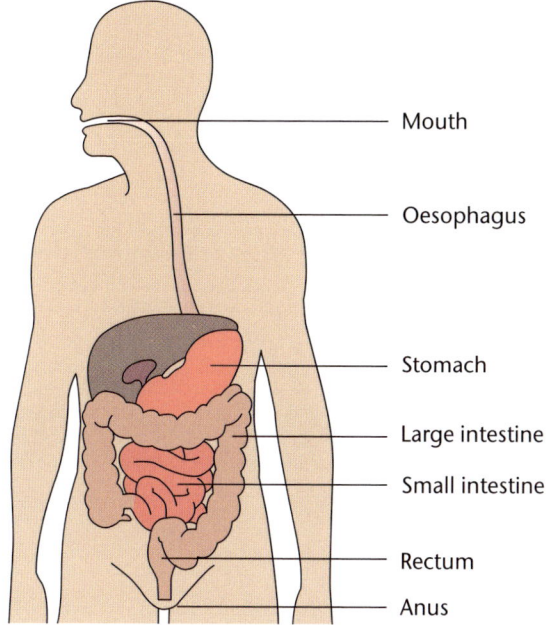

- Mouth
- Oesophagus
- Stomach
- Large intestine
- Small intestine
- Rectum
- Anus

Here is a step-by-step description of what happens to food once it enters your body.

Mouth

Your mouth is a well-known part of the digestive system, the place where food enters the body.

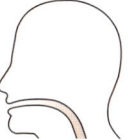

What is going on?
It is in the mouth that a very important thing happens: CHEWING! One of the main reasons you have teeth is to break down the food you eat into smaller parts (known as mechanical digestion), so that when it passes from the mouth to the next stage of the digestive system (to the stomach via the oesophagus) it is easier for your body to deal with. While food is in your mouth it is mixed

with saliva to make it easier to swallow, and saliva also contains an enzyme which starts the breakdown of carbohydrate.

What can go wrong?

With the fast pace of the modern world, people eating and talking at the same time, eating on the run, in the car, or while doing other things, it seems we have lost the art of good old chewing. If you are basically gobbling your food with only the odd chew on the way down, how do you expect your poor old digestive system to cope with massive lumps of food when what it was hoping for was nicely chewed food which it can get to work on digesting?

There are people who say chew your food 20 times, some say 30 times . . . others say chew it until it has no texture; really, it will depend on what you are eating, but my advice is, for goodness' sake, chew your food more than you currently do. Put your knife and fork down between mouthfuls, be mindful of eating slowly and enjoying the taste of your food. Don't be surprised if you are suffering from indigestion, bloating and other digestive problems if you aren't getting this first phase of digestion right.

Oesophagus

From the mouth, your food (well chewed, I hope!) travels down a muscular tube called the oesophagus, which is around 25 cm long. The oesophagus is repeatedly contracting and relaxing to push food down into the stomach.

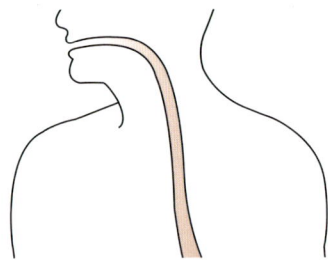

Stomach

Food arrives at the stomach after being pushed down the oesophagus.

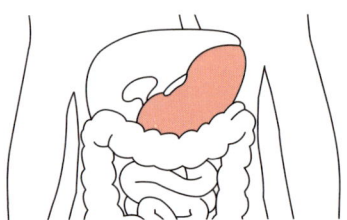

What is going on?

When empty, the stomach is about the size of a clenched fist or a large sausage. It is basically a bag which has some very important jobs to do when it comes to the digestion process – mainly breaking down food into even smaller parts. These jobs are:

1. Producing gastric juice (around 2–3 litres per day in fact), which is a mixture of secretions that helps with the next stage of digestion, breaking down the food you have swallowed. Gastric juice includes:
    *   enzymes to break down protein and fat into smaller parts
    *   hydrochloric acid, also needed to help break down food into small pieces
    *   intrinsic factor, needed for the absorption of vitamin B12.
2. Being a mixing vessel. The stomach allows your food to mix round with gastric juices to break your food into smaller parts.
3. Allowing alcohol to be absorbed into the blood – but no food yet!

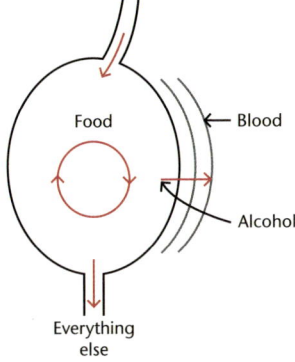

Even though the stomach starts off at the size of a small fist, you will well know that it can hold more food than that. The stomach has the ability to stretch and hold a lot of food if it needs to. When food enters the stomach, it starts to stretch the stomach wall. Over time, the brain is sent a message to tell your body to stop eating because your body has had enough food. An important thing to know, though, is that the feeling of having had enough to eat, being 'full' or satisfied, isn't instant. It can take around 20 minutes for your brain to get up to speed with what you have been eating and realise that you don't need to eat any more! What this means in a practical sense is that if you eat really fast and finish a meal within a few minutes, you may still feel like you need something else to eat and have room for seconds, whereas if you waited another 20 minutes or so after your first serving you would realise that you have actually had enough to eat.

Note to self: eat slowly and wait before having seconds or thinking that you NEED something sweet after your meals!

What can go wrong?

- **Ulcers:** these can form in the stomach as a result of too much acid, taking certain medications or from the presence of a bacteria called *Helicobacter pylori*; the best treatment needs to be discussed with your doctor.
- **Stomach pH:** for digestion to happen properly, it relies on the levels of acidity and alkalinity (measured on the pH scale) to be at an optimum in different parts of the digestive system. The stomach needs to have a low pH (acidic) to allow food to be broken down correctly at this stage. For some people, the pH in their stomach is not what it needs to be, which means that digestion may be compromised. This may be a result of an over- or under-production of acid by the stomach, among other things.
- **Reflux:** sometimes food can go back up the oesophagus, creating a burning sensation because of the highly acidic contents of the stomach which irritate the oesophageal wall. This can happen for a number of reasons, including a problem with the valve at the top of the stomach, which can be made worse by alcohol and smoking.

Small intestine

Hurray – the food has finally been mashed up enough for your body to start putting it to good use, absorbing what it needs and distributing nutrients around the body.

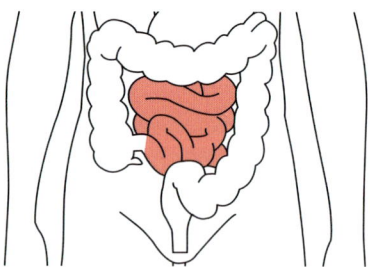

What is going on?

Within two to four hours after eating a meal (depending on what you had and how much), the stomach will start slowly emptying its contents into the small intestine, which is a long wiggly tube about 3 m long.

At the top of the small intestine, the pancreas plays its part by adding pancreatic juice to the digested food, 1.2–1.5 litres per day in fact. This juice changes the pH from acidic to alkaline and adds a whole bunch of enzymes to further assist with the breakdown of carbohydrate, protein and fat. The liver and gall-bladder also have their roles to play, adding bile to the food which, in one of their most important tasks, helps break down fat. On top of this the intestine itself produces even more juices to mix things up.

Once these final digestive juices have been added, it's time to get some work going on . . . this is moving the nutrients (the sugars, amino acids, fatty acids, vitamins and minerals) out of the gut into the blood and lymphatic system to allow them to be transported around the body so they can be used.

The small intestine, as well as being very long, has a massive surface area as it is covered in finger-like projections called villi. As the chewed, mashed and digested food passes over these villi, it can then pass into the blood and lymphatic system – a very, very clever process. Some water is also reabsorbed here.

I hope you can now see the value of a) chewing your food, and b) eating the right things. To allow your body to work at its best, supplying the right types of fuel is essential to keep everything working properly. Your body is relying on you to put the right food in your mouth! In the modern world, where we are surrounded by junk, cheap convenience foods and fizzy drinks, it seems okay to eat them just because they are there. But never forget, just because it is socially normal and acceptable to eat like this, PLEASE do not assume that this is what your body needs. What many people commonly eat these days is based on what they have become accustomed to, what is sold in the shops and what we have developed a taste for – nothing to do with what best supports optimal body function!

Another really important point not to be missed is keeping your intestines healthy to allow your body to absorb the nutrients that you are providing it with.

- **Maintain a healthy balance of bacteria in your gut.** Your gut is full of bacteria, some good and some bad. It is absolutely essential for good health and wellbeing to make sure you have more of the good bacteria and less of the bad. There is a small amount of bacteria in the stomach, a moderate amount in the small intestine and a huge amount in the large intestine, which we will come to next. Probiotics are live microorganisms (bacteria) which can help improve the health of your gut and most people could benefit from including more of these healthy bacteria every day. Ideally, you are looking for a combination of lactobacillus and bifidus bacteria. Probiotics are found in some yoghurts and fermented milk drinks (such as Yakult). For some people, it is also worth considering a good-quality probiotic supplement to get a daily dose of these healthy bacteria. You can get these from any pharmacy, but as with most things, it is worth getting some individual advice on what would suit you best.
- **Keep things flowing.** It is important for digested food and waste to keep moving through your gut so it doesn't end up hanging around inside for too long. If you aren't going to the toilet regularly, this needs to be addressed. Everyone is different, but if it is less than once a day or every second day, you may need to look at your fluid intake, fibre, the balance of bacteria in your gut or something else. Call us at Mission Nutrition to get this sorted – it is not okay to be bunged up!

What can go wrong?

Gosh, where to start? Here are a few common things which can go wrong:

1. **Coeliac disease:** this is an auto-immune disease where eating gluten damages the villi in the small intestine by flattening them. This means that the nutrients from food are then not absorbed properly. The only way to manage this condition is a lifelong gluten-free diet. Coeliac disease is thought to affect one in 100 people in New Zealand and it is diagnosed by a blood test and a positive biopsy (following a colonoscopy). Coeliac disease, however, is NOT the same as gluten intolerance. Eliminating gluten seems to be increasingly popular and although some people are following a gluten-free diet for good reason, there are others who really don't need to be going to such extremes. If you think you have an issue with gluten my recommendation is to seek the advice of your GP or a qualified dietitian/nutritionist who can send you for the right test and ensure you get the best advice. For more on coeliac disease, check out www.coeliac.org.nz.

2. **Lactose intolerance:** the lactase enzyme which breaks down lactose, or milk sugar, sits in the top of the villi. Some people will always be lactose intolerant as they will always be deficient in the lactase enzyme. Others, however, may only have a temporary issue with lactose. If you have had a bout of food poisoning, the gut lining may be damaged and you may be making inadequate amounts of lactase which can cause you to be temporarily lactose intolerant. The same can happen when you are on certain antibiotics. The good news with temporary lactose intolerance is your body can build up its tolerance to lactose over time, and probiotics may also help.

Large intestine

The large intestine or colon is a large tube around 1.5 m long which connects the small intestine to the anus (or bum).

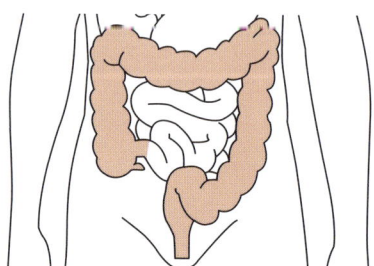

What is going on?

The main jobs of the large intestine are to finish the absorption of nutrients and water from your food and to create the waste product we know all too well as poo.

The final stage of digestion, which is completed in the large intestine, is done by bacteria – these ferment any remaining carbohydrate and produce 'gas' – which we all know exists, whether you are someone who owns up to it or not! It is perfectly normal to pass gas; the issues come when it is in large volumes or very smelly – meaning it is time to address what is going on. As well as fermenting carbohydrate, any remaining protein is broken down. After everything possible has been absorbed, or been transported back to the liver to be dealt with, what remains is poo – a combination of food waste, bacteria and cells which have been shed from the gut lining which is then passed out . . . process complete.

What can go wrong?

1. **Diverticulitis disease:** this is when you get little pockets in the wall of the colon which are called diverticula. Many people who have this will have no symptoms at all; others will develop an inflammation known as diverticulitis, which may cause pain, constipation or the need for frequent trips to the bathroom, nausea and vomiting. Best to seek individual dietary advice if you have this issue.

2. **Ulcerative colitis:** this is a type of inflammatory bowel disease where a layer of the colon or rectum can be inflamed and can result in problems such as a significant change in bowel habits, abdominal pain and loss of blood through the stool. A trip to the doctor and dietary modification is required.

What other issues are common with the digestion process?

Constipation

This is hard stools that are difficult to pass, which may be caused by in-adequate fibre and/or fluid. As I have said before, if this is an issue for you, speak to someone about it. It's not okay to live with this – lots can be done.

Diarrhoea

This is loose unformed stools. A short-term issue could be related to food poisoning, an infection or something similar. If this becomes an on-going issue you will need to head to the doctor to check you don't have irritable bowel syndrome, inflammatory bowel disease, coeliac disease or some other prob-lem – again, best to get it looked into.

Crohn's disease

This is a form of inflammation which can happen in any part of the GI tract and extends through many layers of the gut lining. This can cause pain, issues with malabsorption and in some severe cases requires the removal of the affected part of the gut.

Irritable bowel syndrome (IBS)

Increasingly these days I am seeing people who have issues with pain on eating, bloating, excessive wind and general discomfort. Initially with IBS, I look at the amount of fibre, fluid, fat, spicy food and caffeine someone is having, as these things can all have an impact on gut function. From here, I assess whether any other dietary modification is required. Interesting new research also suggests that there are certain fruits, vegetables and other foods which can cause issues for people with IBS; these foods are collectively known as FODMAPs which stands for fermentable, oligosaccharides, disaccharides, monosaccharaides and polyols. The balance of bacteria in the gut also needs to be considered. For more on this, talk to us at Mission Nutrition (www.missionnutrition.co.nz).

So, overall, you can see that it's not just what you put in your mouth that matters, but also how your body deals with it.

Here are the things you really need to remember:

- Chew your food well.
- Allow 20 minutes after a meal for your brain to register that you have eaten.
- Have plenty of fibre and fluid.
- Be sure to get a good balance of bacteria in your gut.
- If your bowel habits significantly change or you suffer from bloating, excessive wind or abdominal pain, seek medical advice before trying too many random diets!

Part 5: Eat what your body needs

As you know by now, my goal is to help you to understand how to eat what your body needs and how to overcome any practical challenges and difficulties which stand in the way of you eating what you know is good for you.

So, how can you work out exactly what you need to eat to be healthy? Well, that is a good question!

There are so many different ways that people approach this. In the past you may have been given lists of foods that are good and bad. You may have seen food plate models, food pyramids, pages of so-called super foods and foods to avoid. In my opinion, none of these tools actually helps you to practically work out what foods you need to eat during the day to keep your body working at its best.

CATEGORISING FOODS

There are two ways of looking at food when it comes to its nutritional value.

First, you can do it by categorising foods according to the nutrients they contain (nutrients are the building blocks of food, as discussed on page 60). That is, putting together foods high in carbohydrate, those high in protein and those high in fat. The difficulty with this approach is that foods don't normally just contain one nutrient; if you think about pasta, which would be categorised as a carbohydrate, it also has 10 per cent protein, so it really is a mixed food. The same would go for a slice of cheese, considered mainly a protein but over 30 per cent of the slice is fat.

The second way we can look at food is to consider the overall nutritional balance of foods and then 'group' them together if they have a similar nutritional profile. For example, breads and cereals are examples of a food group. Foods within this group are generally very good sources of carbohydrate and provide fibre as well as similar vitamins and minerals. In the same way, milk, yoghurt and cheese can be grouped together – these are all high in protein, have calcium in them and are in many other ways nutritionally similar. It is this approach that is commonly used in New Zealand to provide guidance on what we need to be eating daily for good health, and it is possible to make recommendations on how much we need to eat of each 'group' of food to get the balance of nutrients we need to make our bodies work well.

BUILD YOURSELF A HEALTHY DAY

As useful as it is to understand carbs, protein and fat – the different nutrients – and to have a rough feel for how many grams of each your body needs each day, the reality is that if you were to solely rely on this approach to work out what you should eat for your next meal, you would have to have a calculator at hand all day. Who wants to live like that?

In this book we have used the concept of 'food groups' to create daily food planners and meal ideas for you. Not only will this make it easier to follow, but it is much more straightforward to work out whether you are on target when it comes to getting in the right balance of nutrients you need each day.

DAILY CHECKLIST

For most adults, this is a good guide to what you need to be eating each and every day to help your body function at its best:

Fruit	2 servings a day*
Non-starchy vegetables	3+ servings a day*
Starchy foods	Small amounts at each meal, preferably foods which have been minimally processed
Dairy products, including milk, yoghurt and cheese	2–3 servings a day*
Lean meat, poultry, fish, seafood, eggs and legumes	1–2 servings a day*
Fats and oils	Small amounts of healthy fats
Water	Plenty!

*A serving is roughly what fits into the palm of your hand.

By eating this combination of foods each day, your body will have what it needs to work well: it will supply the right amount of carbohydrate to your brain, the right amount of protein to your muscles and a healthy balance of vitamins and minerals to every cell in your body.

Within each food group you do, however, need to be looking for the healthier option if your goal is weight loss. Let's say you are looking at eating around 6000 kJ a day and you blow 2800 kJ of this on a piece of battered fish and chips; it's going to be pretty tricky to get the remaining food that you need for good health when you only have 3200 kJ to spare! The other thing to remember is that the exact amount you need to eat will vary depending on age and stage, and some of you may have medical conditions or health situations which means this will need to be adapted.

FRUIT

Aim for 2 servings a day. 1 serving is: 1 medium-sized apple, orange or pear, 1 large or 2 small kiwifruit or plums, 1 large slice of pineapple or ½ cup of chopped or canned or stewed fruit.

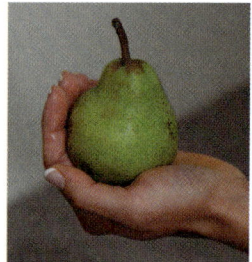 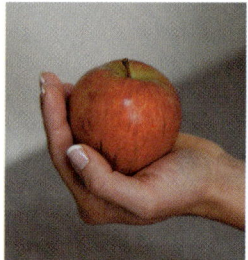 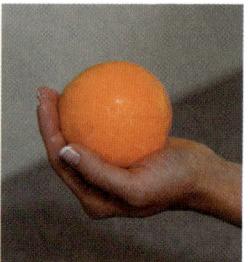

Lose Weight for Life favourites!

As with most things nutrition-related, depending on what you read and who you talk to, you will get different advice on fruit: some are referred to as 'super fruits', others I have seen on 'best to limit' lists. The truth is that fruit does vary: some have higher levels of certain vitamins, minerals, antioxidants and phytochemicals than others and some have a higher GI than others, meaning they make your blood sugars rise more quickly. But as with everything I have said so far, think bigger picture when it comes to fruit.

The best thing you can do for your body is to eat a variety of different fruits to get a mix of the different nutritional goodies. It can be easy to get into the routine of always eating the same few fruits: apples, oranges, bananas . . . so do mix it up!

Here are some ideas for getting more fruit into your diet:

✓   Try using frozen berries or raspberries in a smoothie or on cereal.
✓   Kiwifruit is great to get things moving in your gut, and fab on cereal, in a smoothie or by itself.

✓ Cherries, peaches and nectarines – their season might be short but they just taste fabulous.

✓ Apples and pears grated or finely chopped on top of porridge or Bircher muesli with a sprinkle of cinnamon or mixed spice.

It is always best to eat fruit as fresh as possible and in season is ideal; this maximises the nutritional value of the fruit you are eating. Grow your own where you can – it can save you money and means you can eat fresh every day. I have apples, pears, lemons, limes, feijoas, figs, grapes and strawberries, with raspberries as my latest addition! Frozen fruit can be great, too.

Be mindful

You can have too much of a good thing. If you are having more than three or four pieces of fruit a day (unless you are super active) there may be other important foods you are missing out on. Are you having enough dairy? Enough green veggies? Enough whole grains? I have met many women who definitely eat too much fruit and struggle with their weight because they are just getting too many kilojoules from the one place without balancing everything else out.

As fruit is high in sugar, it is best for you to spread it throughout the day rather than sitting down and eating, say, a whole bunch of grapes in one go – grapes, by the way, have more kilojoules than you may realise and more sugar than your body likes to deal with in one go . . . and may have you heading for the loo later on!

VEGETABLES

The current stats in New Zealand (from the National Nutrition Survey) indicate that around 45 per cent of adults (with men being worse than women) report that they do not have the minimum recommendation of 3 servings of veggies each day.

What is a serving?

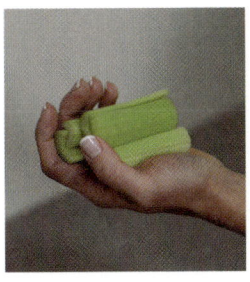 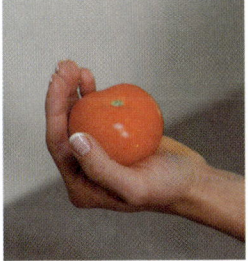 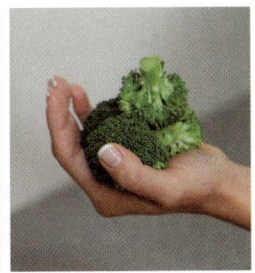

You will have noticed with the well-known 5+ A Day campaign that the plus sign is there, indicating that 5 servings of fruit and veg a day is actually the minimum we need to eat in order to keep well. Really, when it comes to veggies, we are looking at trying to get at least 3+ servings a day. I couldn't agree more . . . go vegetables!

Some people are definitely better than others at meeting the veggie target, but even when I have asked the super-health-conscious to look at how much veg they eat in a week, they aren't eating as many servings as they think. Once you include weekend days, where things tend to be slightly less organised, as well as busy days of the week, veggie consumption can go down.

From my own experience, getting at LEAST 3 handfuls of veggies in each and every day (including weekends) takes some practice and hard work – but, BOY, is it worth it. You do need to look at ways to make veggies part of your daily habits. This has involved me growing my own, using frozen as well as fresh and making use of all parts of the vegetable (that includes broccoli and cauliflower stalks!) to make it financially possible.

Are all vegetables the same?

Well, this is a great one to debate. Other than varying colours and amounts of specific vitamins and minerals in different vegetables, one of the marked differences is the carbohydrate content. This has led to the categorisation of starchy vegetables (potatoes, kumara, yams, taro, green bananas and corn) – which sit at between 15 and 30 per cent carbohydrate – and then the rest which are considered non-starchy. The difference is basically that the starchy vegetables are very high in carbohydrate and the others are lower; although they are all technically vegetables, this massive difference in carbohydrate content means that they do vary considerably from a nutritional point of view. There appears to be no clear cut-off point for the division into starchy and non-starchy and some people will consider vegetables such as parsnip at 11 per cent carbohydrate and pumpkin at 6 per cent as starchy. As a comparison, broccoli is only 2 per cent carbohydrate and tomatoes around 3 per cent.

Without getting too bogged down in the details, the key thing to keep in mind here is that vegetables do vary. Currently the Ministry of Health puts all vegetables in the same category which, although technically correct, does mean that someone who is eating only potatoes, kumara and yams may end up overdoing it on the carbohydrate front and also missing out on the nutritional goodness of greens or the other great colour-packed, non-starchy vegetables. In this book we will be considering the higher starch vegetables separately and putting potatoes, kumara, yams, taro, green bananas and corn in with other starchy foods such as breads and cereals.

Lose Weight for Life favourites!

✓ Aim for at LEAST 3 servings (big handfuls) of non-starchy veggies a day – more is better.

✓ Go for plenty of green veggies – spinach, silver beet, cabbage, kale, pak choy, broccoli – they have a fabulous number of vitamins and minerals.

✓ Use as little water as possible when cooking your vegetables and don't overcook them – some of the vitamins are water-soluble, which means that they get lost and thrown away in the cooking water.

✓ Include raw veggies as well as cooked – some vitamins are destroyed by heat and light – so pick fresh, and eat fresh.

✓ Try planting spinach, silver beet, salad greens and rocket – they are super easy to grow. You can get miniature versions, too, called micro greens, which are great in salads.

✓ Beetroot and other purple veggies often get forgotten. Include a variety of colours to get a variety of nutrients – go wild!

✓ Have a handful of veggies at lunch, a vegetable snack and then veggies at dinner EVERY DAY to get your quota.

✓ See the recipe section at the back of the book to get more ideas for great ways to eat more veggies.

STARCHY FOODS

The starchy food group includes bread, crackers, rice, pasta, cereals and other grain-based products – this is also where I like to put potatoes, kumara, yams, taro, green bananas and corn, as previously mentioned, given that they have a high proportion of starch compared with other vegetables. These foods essentially provide a good dose of carbohydrate, but depending on the type you choose, can either provide next to no other nutritional goodness (that's your heavily processed grains!) or a WHOLE massive heap of goodies (go whole grains!).

How much do you need?

The foods in this group provide lots of carbohydrate, some fibre and a range of vitamins and minerals. The amount that you need varies hugely depending on how active you are – the more active you are, the more you are likely to need. As a general rule, though, for most people I suggest including some form of fabulously healthy carbohydrate at each meal and if you are active, with your snacks, too. For someone watching their waistline this may be anything from say $1/3$–$1/2$ cup of wholegrain oats for breakfast, $1/2$–$3/4$ cup of cooked brown rice at lunch and $1/2$–$3/4$ cup of cooked quinoa or a small baked kumara at dinner. If I was working with someone who was super active and not needing to lose much weight, it could be that they would need 1–2 cups of starchy foods at each meal – it does depend on who you are and what your goals are.

Does it matter what time you eat these foods if you are watching your weight?

Your body is burning carbohydrate at all times, as it is the source of fuel your brain is using – and your brain is busy working away 24 hours a day, yes, even when you are sleeping. So even if you are trying to lose weight, having small amounts of starchy foods at each meal is fine provided these foods are included as part of your total daily kilojoule budget.

Your body burns additional carbohydrate when you are active, running, briskly walking, at gym classes, so it is logical to include more carbohydrate on the days when you are most active. Practically, this means that if you are really busy all morning, running around, exercising first thing, you will definitely need a dose of carbs at breakfast and lunch. If you were then to go home and sit on the sofa all evening or spend most of the night sitting down, it would be okay to have less carbs with your evening meal. The opposite also applies.

If you fall into work having taken three steps from your car and sit at your desk all day long, less of your carbohydrate allowance would be needed at this part of the day. If you then head to the gym after work, for a run or are busy and active all evening, the really important times for you to be having more carbs would be at afternoon tea to fuel you for your workout and at dinner to help your body recover.

As with so many aspects of nutrition, and despite the love of rules, lists and ideals, one size does not fit all.

Lose Weight for Life favourites!

These are the starchy carbs which are less processed, high in fibre, with the maximum number of nutrients and higher in B vitamins which people can be short on. My top picks:

- ✓ Brown rice
- ✓ Oats
- ✓ Rye
- ✓ Barley
- ✓ Buckwheat
- ✓ Spelt
- ✓ Quinoa.

Other foods you can include:

- ✓ Dense wholegrain breads and pumpernickel
- ✓ Wholegrain crackers
- ✓ Baked or boiled potato, kumara and yams – leave the skin on for extra fibre
- ✓ Taro, green bananas – be mindful of portions, though
- ✓ Basmati rice – yes, it is white, but it has a low GI so is fine to use for variety
- ✓ Pasta – despite being white in appearance, it still has a low GI.

Least nutritionally valuable, heavily processed grains:

- ✓ White bagels, white bread and white wraps
- ✓ Cakes, biscuits and scones made totally from white flour.

Why are some people carb-phobic?

Over the last five years or so there has been a re-emergence of carb phobia. You know what I mean: don't eat carbs at night, avoid all bread, cut down on grains – and this is an increasingly controversial area of nutrition.

There is no denying that if you combed through your diet and ate exactly the same as you do now but minus a lot of the carbs, you would lose weight – of course you would. First, by doing this, you would be cutting at least a few hundred kilojoules out of your diet; and second, when you cut out carbs, your body depletes its carbohydrate stores (called glycogen) and, in the process of doing this, loses water at the same time – meaning you may see a nice shift down in the number of kilos on the scales.

Sounds like the perfect idea, and I do get that, but . . . it really isn't, and I would never put myself through it. Although in the short term you can lose weight, after a while cravings can emerge. From what I have seen, people get desperate for sugary lollies, cakes, biscuits, really anything sweet, and this can start the terrible restriction-and-binge cycle – hello emotional eating! The other thing is that when you drop your carbohydrate intake too low, you can find it hard to think and concentrate, and exercising can become very difficult as you will feel tired and fatigued very quickly. On top of this you are at risk of not getting the value from other nutrients such as fibre and B vitamins, which come along with the whole grains and healthy starchy foods.

The worst part of it all is that if you have restricted your carbs and then have a day when you think 'Sod it, I am eating a sandwich and pasta', then your weight can sky-rocket by a few kilos in just a day. This can make you think that the carbs have made you gain weight super fast, but this is just not the case. This is your body holding on to some water again with the re-introduction of carbs; if you don't understand this, it only adds to the mistaken conclusion that carbs make you fat.

Now, I am not for one second suggesting you start digging into the bagels, white toast or endless bowls of pasta with creamy sauces, but it is really about acknowledging that, with a long-term goal of maintaining good health and a healthy weight, including some carbohydrate-rich foods is helpful. If you are carrying a lot more weight than is healthy and/or you are not able to be very active, you will certainly need less than someone busy and active, but it is a case of striking the balance of what is right for you.

DAIRY PRODUCTS, INCLUDING MILK, YOGHURT AND CHEESE

Some people really enjoy drinking milk, love the taste of yoghurt and can't go past a slice of cheese or three (particularly if it is with crackers and wine); there are others who aren't quite so hot on the dairy front. This is a really important food group to think about when it comes to your health and wellbeing, so it is good to know where you stand and if you are getting what your body needs.

Dairy products provide protein, but also, very importantly, calcium as well as a range of other nutritional wonders.

For those who are allergic to or intolerant of cow's milk and associated products, luckily there are lots of good alternatives on the market now, including soy milks as well as fortified milks made from rice and oats.

How much do you need?

It is recommended that adults include 2–3 servings of dairy a day and that post-menopausal women need 4 servings a day as their need for calcium increases with the changes in hormone levels. A serving is 1 cup of milk, 2 slices of cheese or 1 pottle of yoghurt.

Most New Zealanders over 15 years of age aren't getting enough calcium, so this is a food group most people need to focus on, because – think about it – do you get 2–3 servings of dairy a day?

Lose Weight for Life favourites!

- ✓ Low-fat milks including trim, super trim and calcium-enriched trim milk. These milks are appropriate for most adults, with the calcium-enriched versions being particularly beneficial for women who have higher calcium needs at certain stages of life.
- ✓ Cheeses vary hugely in their fat content. Edam is a lower-fat hard cheese, but is still 25 per cent fat so isn't good to go wild with.
- ✓ Ricotta is a great replacement for creamy pasta sauces or on wholegrain crackers – and, a bonus, you can buy reduced-fat varieties, too.
- ✓ Cottage cheese is excellent. It is a fabulous source of protein and low in kilojoules, but do be aware, it contains very little calcium.
- ✓ Yoghurt – unsweetened, low-fat natural varieties are my favourite. You can make your own with a yoghurt maker if you prefer. Add fruit for sweetness.

Be mindful

There are some yoghurts that have a huge amount of sugar, some of which will be from the milk (lactose), but many varieties will also have lots of added sugar. For when you are reading labels, a helpful tip is: 4 g = 1 teaspoon of sugar.

There are lots of creamy 'posh' yoghurts on the market at the moment and some of them are incredibly high in fat. Something over 5 per cent fat (i.e. more than 5 g in 100 g) is really very high for a yoghurt – I have seen some up to 10 g per 100 g. Let's take something in the middle at say 7 g in 100 g: that would mean that in a small pot (150 g) you would be having over 10 g of fat – that is 2 teaspoons' worth!

It can be easy to overdo the cheese, and the blues, bries and tastys of this world really are the high-kilojoule traps within this food group. It's best not to nibble on cheese if you are trying to lose weight – grate it or use it as an ingredient in cooking. You can get away with using a lot less if you use a small amount of a cheese with a strong flavour, too.

MEAT, FISH AND PROTEIN ALTERNATIVES

In New Zealand you can buy an array of delicious and tasty meats, poultry, fish, seafood, eggs and alternative sources of protein. From a nutritional standpoint there are so many fabulous things to say about these foods; the key is getting the right balance of each type. (That's if you aren't vegetarian or vegan – more on this later!)

Red meat

A fabulous source of protein, iron, zinc and the B group vitamins. The World Cancer Research Fund suggests limiting meat to around 750 g raw meat (around 500 g cooked) per week. If you consider that a palm-sized piece of meat (I emphasise PALM, not your hand!) is around 150 g, you should be eating this amount no more than five times a week. Remember, this is the maximum recommended, not a goal to aim for. Nutrition- and cost-wise, eating meat two to three times a week is totally sufficient, and I certainly don't have more than this. Remember to trim all the extra fat off meat.

Fish

Another incredible source of protein. Fish with a lower fat content are mainly white fish such as snapper, John Dory and hoki. There are also oilier varieties like salmon, trout, sardines and mackerel, which have far more fat. This is good news for once, though; the fat in these fish is very good for you because it is packed with lots of omega 3. Aim to eat fish at LEAST 2–3 times a week if possible, with 1–2 servings of oily fish. To make this affordable, buy what is on special, and there are some cheaper types of fish which might not be great to have on their own but are lovely in a curry or in a pie. Frozen fish is a good alternative, too.

Omega 3

Long-chain omega 3 fatty acids are known as essential fats – this is because your body is unable to make them by itself so you need to get these through your diet. These fatty acids are important at every stage of life. During pregnancy they help with the development and healthy growth of a baby's brain, eyes and nervous system. The need for omega 3 carries on for children and adults of all ages to continue keeping the brain healthy and functioning at its best throughout life.

Omega 3 fats are important to maintain a healthy heart, not to mention keeping your bones and joints in good condition. The recommended intake of long-chain omega 3 fatty acids per day to help promote good health and prevent chronic diseases is 610 mg for men and 430 mg for women. The specific type of long-chain omega 3 fatty acids that you are looking for are called DHA and EPA, and the combined amount of these two needs to add up to the recommended totals.

Salmon is by far the richest source of these fatty acids; if you eat a 150 g serving of salmon once a week you will be on target for what you need, and

2 servings a week would be even better. My recommendation is to always make sure you buy New Zealand king salmon rather than other imported varieties such as Atlantic salmon. King salmon has far more of these long-chain omega 3 fats than the other types. For more on salmon, check out www.regalsalmon. co.nz, which has some great information on king salmon and some excellent recipes, too.

Other good sources of long-chain omega 3 fatty acids include sardines, trout and mackerel. White fish and other seafood such as oysters, scallops and prawns also contain some omega 3.

There is a second type of omega 3 fatty acid known as short-chain omega 3 or ALA. This is found in flaxseeds (or linseeds), walnuts and chia seeds. These are certainly good for your health, but don't have the same health benefits associated with the long-chain variety. A small amount of the short-chain fatty acid is converted into long-chain fatty acid in the body, but not a huge amount so it will still be important to include sources of long-chain omega 3 fatty acid as well. For more on this, head to www.omega-3centre.com.

Eggs

Eggs can make a great breakfast, lunch, dinner or snack. There is no single guideline around the number of eggs that is okay for the average person to eat; however, if you do have high cholesterol it is recommended to limit the number of eggs you have. For more information on this, see www.heartfoundation.org.nz.

Alternatives

For vegetarians and non-vegetarians, there is huge value in including alternative sources of protein such as tofu (which has all the essential amino acids – yay!), lentils, chickpeas, kidney beans, butter beans and haricot beans.

For non-vegetarians, I suggest aiming for 1–2 vegetarian meals a week – they can be much cheaper and are a nutritional dream.

For vegetarians and vegans, there is a risk that you are not getting enough protein in your diet so it will be important to seek advice to check if you are getting enough and mixing your proteins to get a complete blend (see page 65 on the amount of protein you need). Nuts are also a source of protein and can be helpful for vegetarians and vegans to include, but remember they are very high in kilojoules so portion control is key here.

Lose Weight for Life favourites!

✓ Include a variety of different protein-rich foods in your diet.

✓ Limit red meat to 750 g raw (500 g cooked) a week.

✓ Eat more fish, especially fresh salmon and other oily fish which are packed with omega 3.

✓ Eat vegetarian a few nights a week – it saves money and is good for you, too. Try curries, salads and stews made with pulses, tofu with a stir-fry or go for an omelette packed with vegetables along with a salad on the side.

✓ Use chickpeas, lentils, kidney beans and any other legumes you like in salads, casseroles and soups.

Be mindful

- Processed meats such as salami and pepperoni can be very high in salt as well as saturated fat.
- Have your eggs the healthy way – poached or boiled – and watch what you have on the side. Adding a few spoonfuls of hollandaise on top is like adding a chocolate bar to your meal in terms of the extra fat and energy from the sauce.
- Go easy on the nuts. Half a cup of mixed nuts is 1890 kJ and if you are aiming for the 6000 kJ a day, that is one-third of your day's budget gone!

HEALTHY FAT

As we have seen on page 68, your body does need some healthy fat to function well. It provides energy as well as the fat-soluble vitamins A, D, E and K. Unsaturated fats are best. Fats are incredibly high in energy, so I suggest using smaller quantities of good-quality oils. It is helpful to consider serving sizes of this group. Use a teaspoon rather than a tablespoon of oil when cooking. A single tablespoon is 500 kJ – the same energy as 1½ slices of bread!

Lose Weight for Life favourites!

✓ Extra-virgin olive oil for cooking and flaxseed oil for salads and dressings. Canola and ricebran oils can be good to have at hand, too.

✓ Use avocado as a spread. I've included it here because avocados are 25 per cent fat, with an average avocado at around 40 g fat.

✓ Nuts and seeds, while they do contain some protein, have some healthy fats, too, so I have included them here. They range from 50 to 80 per cent fat.

✓ Nut butters without added salt or sugar – try making your own.

Be mindful

- Consider the amount of fat you have in your meals and snacks. Limit the total fat per meal to around 10–15 g and 5–10 g in a snack. If you sit down and have something like a big biscuit, that's 25 g in one sitting, and it was just a snack.
- Minimise trans-fat and saturated animal fat as much as possible.
- When cooking with oil, measure out what you are using with a teaspoon rather than mindlessly pouring it into the pan – you should hopefully end up using less oil!

WHERE DO DRINKS FIT IN?

Now we have talked about food and what to eat each day, let's look at another hugely important factor – hydration. The majority of the body is made up of water, which plays a number of vital roles such as keeping your blood flowing, regulating your body temperature and allowing your muscles to contract. It is also required in the digestive process to allow food to be broken down and absorbed, and for waste products to be got rid of. You also further lose water every day through urine, sweating and breathing – so it is no surprise that it is super important to make sure you replace what you have lost!

The amount you need to drink is yet another point of debate, with some suggesting you need a certain number of litres each day, and others recommending you have a specific number of glasses or cups. But, boy, have I heard some crazy recommendations in my time. The Ministry of Health guidelines advise that an adequate intake is 2.1 litres for women and 2.6 litres for men – but this is just a starting point.

The reality is there is no exact amount of fluid that works for everyone; it varies depending on how much you sweat, how much you move around and whether you work outside all day or in an air-conditioned office. The ideal amount to drink is the amount which results in you producing large volumes of pale-coloured urine – this is a good indication that you are well hydrated and that your body is getting the fluid that it needs. For most people, they will need to drink more than they are now.

I like using a pee chart when I am talking to people about hydration as it is a great visual indicator of what you need to be looking for.

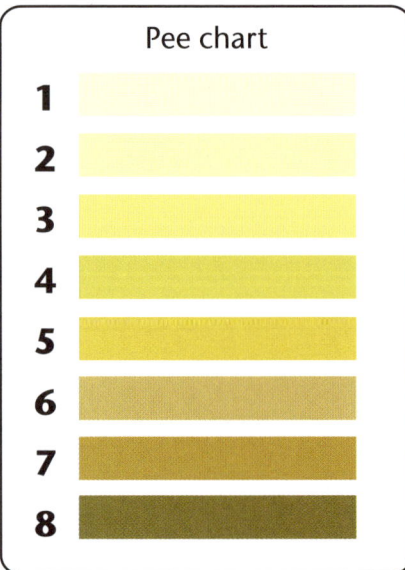

Pee chart

1
2
3
4
5
6
7
8

Your target is to make sure that your pee is the same colour as numbers 1, 2 or 3. Colours 4 and 5 suggest dehydration, and 6 and 7 severe dehydration.

Note that this is a guide only as individual diets will cause slight variations in colour.

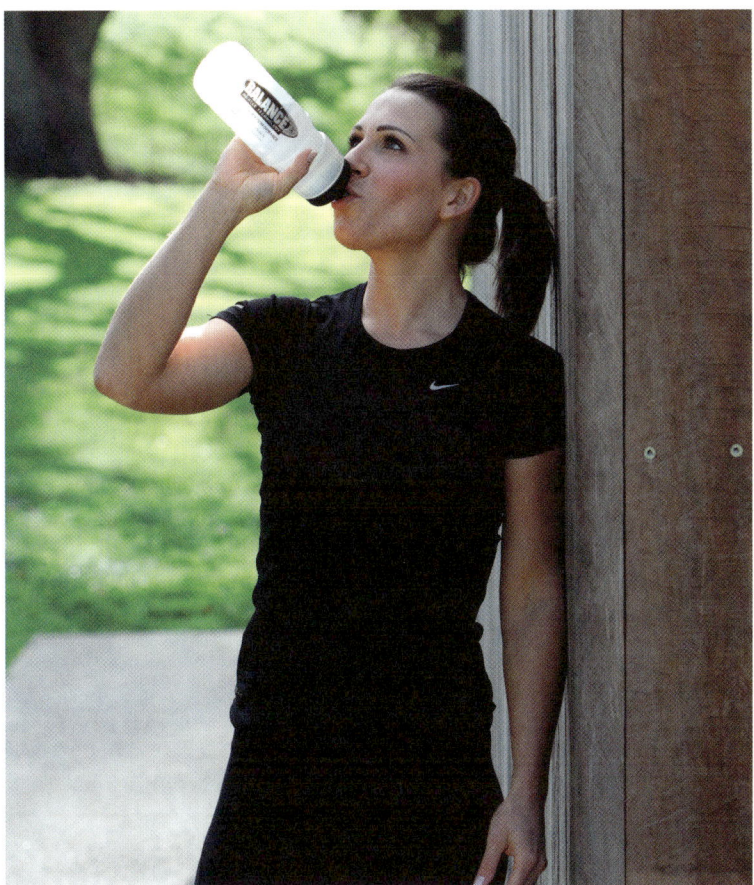

Ideally, aim to be between 1 and 3 on the pee chart during the day. Things may look a little darker when you wake up in the morning, having not drunk overnight, but your pee should soon come back in line after a few glasses of water.

Anything above 3 suggests dehydration and this is not good. Dehydration of as little as a 2 per cent loss of body weight can result in impaired physiological responses and performance – i.e. your brain won't be working so well – so it is worth keeping hydration in mind when it comes to keeping yourself well.

Top tips for hydration

✓ Carry a water bottle with you wherever you go and have two in the fridge at all times so you can grab one as you leave the house for work.

✓ Establish a drinking routine – 2 glasses of water before you leave the house and a glass of water with every meal and snack.
✓ Keep chilled water in the fridge with added mint, sliced lemon, lime or orange for a tasty, healthy refreshment.

There are lots of different things available to drink

- The best everyday choice is water. Try hot water with fresh mint leaves, slices of ginger or lemon.
- Herbal teas and green tea are also great.
- A cup of fruit juice can be counted as 1 fruit serving, but it is still high in sugar so best diluted down; or try a mixed fruit and veggie juice. When you are watching your weight, though, it is better overall to eat your fruit rather than drink it.
- If you do high-intensity or endurance sports, when you are training for several hours at a time sports waters and sports drinks can be helpful – but your average sports drink has 14 teaspoons of sugar and more kilojoules than a chocolate bar. For most of you reading this, I would steer clear.
- Drinks such as coke, Fanta, lemonade, L&P, Red Bull, V, GForce, E2 and others are full of sugar and aren't ideal everyday choices – a total waste of your kilojoule budget and not good for you on so many levels.
- Diet or zero-sugar fizzy drinks are okay occasionally if you choose to include these. They don't contain sugar, but they do contain acid which isn't good for your teeth.

Coffee and tea

How much do some people love their morning coffee? Caffeine has become such a habit for some people that it seems they are gripping onto that take-away cup of latte for dear life, just to ensure they have the mental capacity to walk into the office in the morning! I have seen near-fights between people waiting in line for coffee in the morning when the queues are really long – what's happened to us?

Here is what has happened: in some parts of the country, coffee has become an institution and a craze – these days meetings are over coffee, catching up with friends is over coffee, feeling a bit tired and run down . . . no guesses for what people run for.

A huge number of people that I meet definitely have a strong dependency on coffee; it has become a routine, a ritual, just part of what happens in their day. But the truth is, for some, when you over-do the coffee, you end up worse off – more tired – so you need to strike a balance.

Coffee and tea are an important part of our world; occasionally, you find people who can't stand either and go for the hot chocolate option, but for the rest of us, we enjoy them – some a little, some A LOT.

From a health perspective, most people should have no major concerns with including a couple of cups of tea and/or coffee during the day. It is indeed a mental stimulant and can help you to concentrate better. There are no set guidelines for adults when it comes to caffeine, but I would definitely suggest keeping below 300 mg a day, which seems adequate for most people I work with. In pregnancy it is recommended to limit caffeine to 200 mg a day. Be mindful that some people are also more sensitive to the effects of caffeine than others.

How much caffeine is in your drink?*
- 1 shot (30 ml) of espresso coffee = 65 mg
- 1 teaspoon of instant coffee = 56 mg
- 1 cup of English breakfast tea = 55 mg

Note: these are estimates as the amount varies in different brands.

How does this compare with other caffeinated drinks?
- 1 can of Red Bull (250 ml) = 80 mg
- 1 can of V (250 ml) = 78 mg
- 1 can of cola (355 ml) = 34 mg
- 1 can of Mother energy drink (500 ml) = 160 mg

One thing you do need to consider, however, is that caffeine has a really long half-life. What I mean by that is after you have drunk a cup, it stays in your system for a really long time. In fact, six hours after your morning coffee, there is still around HALF the amount of caffeine in your system. Why does this even matter? Well, caffeine is a stimulant; if you have too much hanging around in your body at night, it affects the quality of your sleep. More on this later . . .

Alcohol

There are positive and negative things about alcohol. There is some evidence to suggest that a few alcoholic drinks a day may decrease the risk of heart disease and stroke in older adults. However, before you get too excited, the Heart Foundation is currently questioning this as a reason to justify drinking alcohol. There are other much healthier ways to improve your heart health without needing to drink.

On the downside – well, we could be here for hours. Drinking alcohol can increase your risk of cancer, and the more you drink, the bigger the risk. Regular drinkers are more likely to get chronic diseases and, in the same way that having caffeine in your system affects your sleep, booze does too. If you are using alcohol to help you sleep, it might knock you out but you are unlikely to feel more rested in the morning.

From a weight point of view, things aren't looking too bright either; alcohol is really high in kilojoules, damn it! If you are really serious about losing weight and keeping it off, as much as I love a great glass of vino or cocktail myself, the truth is that less is better – even if you go for the lower-kilojoule options.

The drinks . . . (average drink sizes)

150 ml wine 520 kJ = 25 min walk	**Double gin & tonic** 960 kJ = 45 min walk	**Double gin & DIET tonic** 525 kJ = 25 min walk
Cosmo (cocktail) 710 kJ = 33 min walk	**RTD (e.g. Smirnoff Ice)** 710 kJ = 33 min walk	**330 ml lager** 565 kJ = 27 min walk
Pina Colada (cocktail) 1255 kJ = 60 min walk	**60 ml Baileys** 710 kJ = 33 min walk	**330 ml low-carb beer** 460 kJ = 22 min walk

When you are watching your waistline, is it better to drink beer or wine?

Sadly, neither. As you will see from the table above, both beer and wine are quite similar in their kilojoules when you consider an average drink size. A 330 ml bottle of a 5 per cent lager-type beer is anywhere from 584 kJ whereas a 150 ml glass of wine (a fifth of a bottle) is around 520 kJ.

There is a common misconception that beer and wine have lots of sugar in them and that is part of the reason why they can cause weight gain. However, this isn't really true. Most beers have less than a teaspoon of sugar in them, similar to a glass of wine (depending on the wine, of course), but this is nothing compared with the 8 teaspoons in a 355 ml can of fizzy drink. The reality is that alcohol itself is very high in kilojoules: 1 g of alcohol is 28 kJ compared with 1 g of sugar which is 16 kJ. So it is the alcohol component in beer and wine that pushes up the kilojoules and makes it very unhelpful for weight loss.

The lower-kilojoule drinks are low-alcohol beers and a single unit (yes, just 30 ml) of a spirit like gin, vodka, or rum with a diet mixer or soda, which is only 266 kJ a serve.

Is low-carb beer a better choice?

It is a common perception that low-carb beers are better for the waistline than standard beers. Truth be known, beer isn't that high in carbs, anyway; a standard lager has no more than 10–15 g per bottle which isn't really that much. Low-carb beers can be very slightly lower in kilojoules than standard beers, but the amount really is quite small and it doesn't mean you can drink beer endlessly. The best beer if you are watching your waistline is a low-alcohol variety. Overall, my advice when it comes to beer is to have less of the beer you enjoy rather than having more of a 'healthier' beer. Less alcohol, all round, is better for you.

Lose Weight for Life advice

✓ Ladies, try to keep your total alcohol intake to 10 units, or less, per week. Men should aim for less than 15 units. This is lower than what you may have been told before, but it is the current advice given by the Alcohol Advisory Council (www.alac.org.nz) to help reduce alcohol-related health risks – given the problems alcohol can cause, I am happy to support drinking less alcohol. A unit of alcohol is 100 ml of wine (12.5% alcohol), 330 ml of beer (4% alcohol) or 30 ml of a spirit (40% alcohol). Be sure to have at least two alcohol-free days each week (ideally more) and avoid having too much alcohol in one sitting – there are serious consequences.

✓ If you are using alcohol to cope with stress or to get you to sleep, we need to find you a new habit. Check out pages 190–92.
✓ If you drink a lot because it is what your friends do and it's a normal habit, this doesn't mean you have to be the boring one. Check out page 192 for strategies.
✓ If you are drinking spirits, make vodka with fresh lime or lemon and soda your drink of choice.
✓ Have fewer beers or go for the lower-alcohol ones.
✓ Top wine with soda and don't keep a bottle of white wine chilled in the fridge 'just in case', or you will drink it because it is there.

Part 6: Total health and wellbeing – keep fit, sleep well

The focus of this book so far has been on nutrition, food and eating (yum yum!) which is no surprise given that this is my primary area of expertise. However, to lose weight, keep it off and live a healthy well-balanced life, it is super important to mention some of the other things which affect your health and wellbeing. Exercise and sleep are the two big ones in my mind. When you combine the power of great nutrition with an active lifestyle and good-quality sleep, you have a winning formula to live a fabulous healthy life and, of course, Lose Weight for Life.

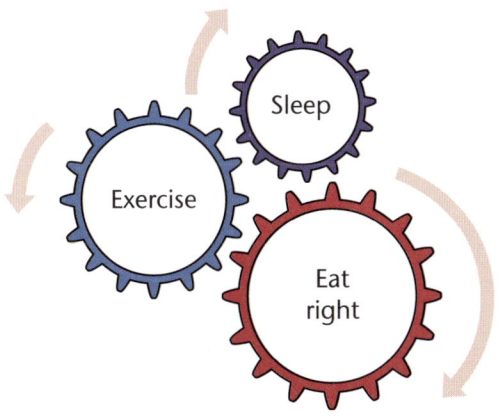

KEEPING FIT

Exercise is a funny thing. Some people find it really easy to motivate themselves to get their trainers on, head out for a walk, run or to a pump class, but
others just want to curl up in a ball with their fingers in their ears when the
word 'exercise' is even mentioned.

Why bother with keeping fit?

At school I always got picked last for the sports teams and was just un-
believably terrible at playing sport. I couldn't run to save my life and got
thrown out of dance classes because I was too chubby (how rude!) and my
co-ordination was just all wrong. Surprisingly, though, later in life, I somehow
managed to regain my confidence with exercise (slowly, I have to add) and
ended up training to become a fitness instructor teaching complicated aerobics moves and dance.

In my early twenties, I spent a few years teaching group-fitness classes and
helping clients one on one in a personal-training job – and I loved it. What I
enjoyed the most was the reward of seeing people over time feel better about
themselves, look better and improve their overall physical and mental health
– all by getting fitter.

Regardless of the fitness level people started with (some couldn't even walk
to the letterbox at the end of their drive without having to stop three times
when I first met them), the positive results were always the same. The other
thing I noticed was that when people started to get fitter and build up their
confidence, they often began to eat better, too, not wanting to binge on rubbish or rely on convenience food – good habits breed good habits.

For you to lose weight, keep it off and live an overall healthy balanced life,
keeping fit is just non-negotiable. To get the results you really want, I can promise
you, as super-mega-important as it is to look at what you are eating and why,
looking at the fitness side of things is also vital. That doesn't mean you need
to get into some super-tight lycra or enter the Ironman tomorrow, but it does
mean that if you aren't currently active, something needs to change. Keeping
fit should be part of your life, not something you do for six weeks or on a 12-
week challenge. It is all about starting somewhere, progressively working on
your overall fitness and making exercise part of your daily routine.

The benefits of being fit

Where to start! The list of benefits is massive and the thing to note from this
list of goodies is that exercise has positive effects on all parts of your life – not
just on your physical body. Exercise:

- ✓ Helps you to maintain a healthy weight – phew!
- ✓ Helps to increase bone density and strength – very important, we
  don't want crumbling bones.
- ✓ Can help to improve your mood and motivation – this is such a
  good reason to get and stay fit.

✓ Can help you to live longer and optimise your quality of life.
✓ Helps to keep your heart strong and working at its best.
✓ Reduces the risks of heart disease, cancer, diabetes, stroke and high blood pressure.
✓ Is a fantastic way to deal with stress.
✓ Improves sleep, which has a knock-on effect to other areas of your life, as we will discuss further on.
✓ Helps to reduce the risk of falls by improving balance and co-ordination, especially useful for older adults.

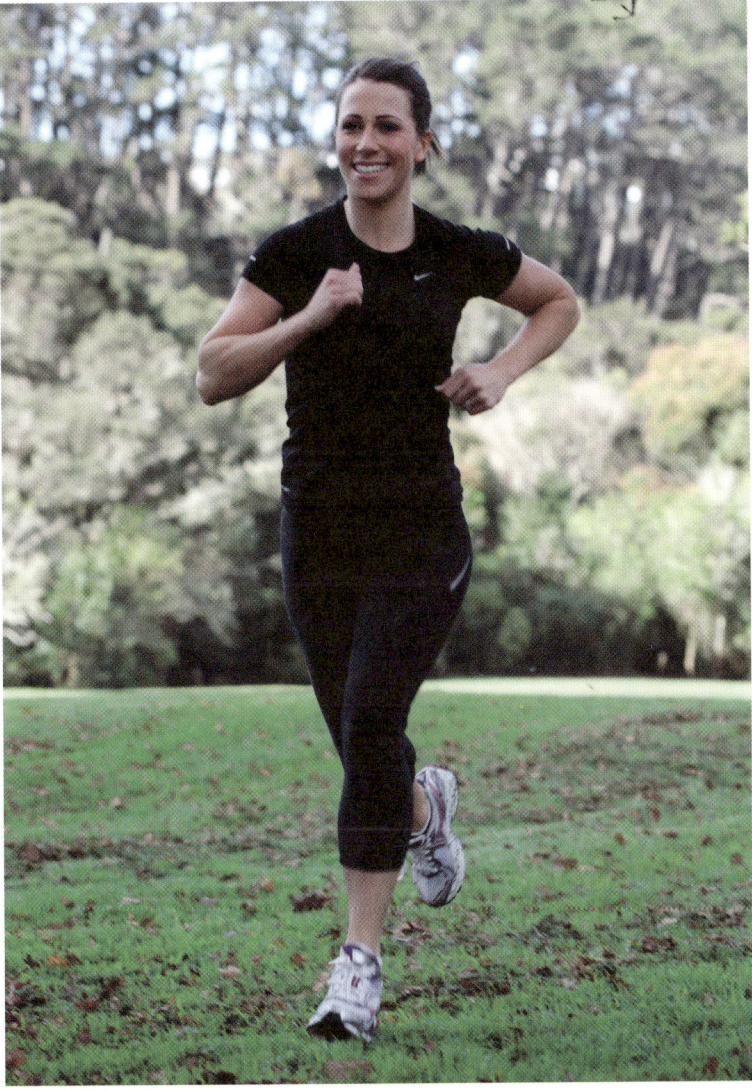

What type of exercise do I need to do to keep fit?

Being fit isn't just about being able to run. It is also about having muscular strength, endurance and flexibility. Ideally, I encourage people to do a variety of exercise to work on all the different components of their fitness – that is the best way to get a good balance.

Cardiovascular exercise

This includes sports and activities such as walking, running, cycling, swimming, rowing, hiking, tennis, boxing, netball, football, rugby, rugby league, touch rugby, athletics and aerobics classes.

Major benefits include:

- Strengthening the heart
- Improving circulation
- Reducing blood pressure.

The key thing here is to get started somewhere, so even if, for now, it is just walking and swimming, that is okay. You can build on this as you go. The important thing is that you aim to get progressively fitter; in my experience people tend to reach a certain level of fitness, get comfortable and stay there. If you can currently comfortably run three times a week, why not make your pace a bit faster, change your running route or add some sprinting into the mix? If you swim slowly a few times a week, add in an aerobics class and a long walk at the weekend – step things up! To get results you need to change things up, as your body will just adapt to what you always do which just makes it much harder to get results.

I am a big fan of adding high-intensity bursts into my exercise regimen – these add a whole new dimension to training and I find I get really good results in increasing fitness and helping with weight loss. Here is how it can work:

WALKING

If you normally go for an hour-long walk, try jogging for a minute after five minutes of walking and repeat this for the entire time you are out. Once you have got this pattern sussed, mix it up some more. Try jogging for two minutes, running for one minute and then walking for 10 minutes – just aim to change the intensity and add some 'bursts' each time.

RUNNING

If you currently run for say 30 minutes, why not add in some small sprints; maybe sprint between every second lamp post you come across. If there are some steps or a hill on your running route, run up and down the steps or the hill a few times to up the intensity.

SWIMMING

Rather than just swimming at a steady pace, every few lengths do one length where you are swimming as fast as you possibly can – go for it! Then repeat this, say every two or three lengths.

Strength or resistance training

This includes things such as free weights, fixed weight machines, pump gym classes, press-ups, squats, lunges, triceps dips and chin-ups.

Major benefits include:

- Increasing muscular strength
- Enhancing bone density
- Increasing metabolic rate.

Never underestimate the benefits of strength and resistance training when it comes to weight loss. Lots of people are very scared of doing weights because they think they will bulk up and look bigger. But if you are getting the right advice and doing the exercises properly, this won't happen.

Muscle is metabolically very active; what that means is that even when muscle is not busy working out (say when you are sitting down doing nothing or asleep), your muscle tissue is still burning lots and lots of kilojoules, whereas fat tissue doesn't. The advantage, therefore, of building up your muscle mass is that you're able to increase your metabolic rate and burn off what you eat more quickly – it doesn't take a rocket scientist to work out that this is a really helpful step in the weight-loss process.

So, I would urge you to consider including some form of strength and resistance training, preferably at least a few times a week. There are some suggested exercise plans on page 120 onwards from a good friend of mine, Dave Margison, who is an excellent trainer.

Flexibility

This includes activities such as yoga, Pilates and stretching.

Major benefits include:

- Preventing injury and pain
- Improving posture
- Improving range of movement.

Can't touch your toes? Legs get really tight and sore after a long walk? Time to get flexible! Don't overlook this as part of a fitness plan – put some stretching into your weekly workout routine.

How much do I need to do?

My suggestion is for you to try to be physically active (over and above your normal daily walking around) at the very least for 30 minutes each day, aiming for an hour and preferably more. This can be done all in one go or you can split your exercise into several bursts throughout the day if it is easier. It all really depends on where you are now, but the goal is over the weeks and

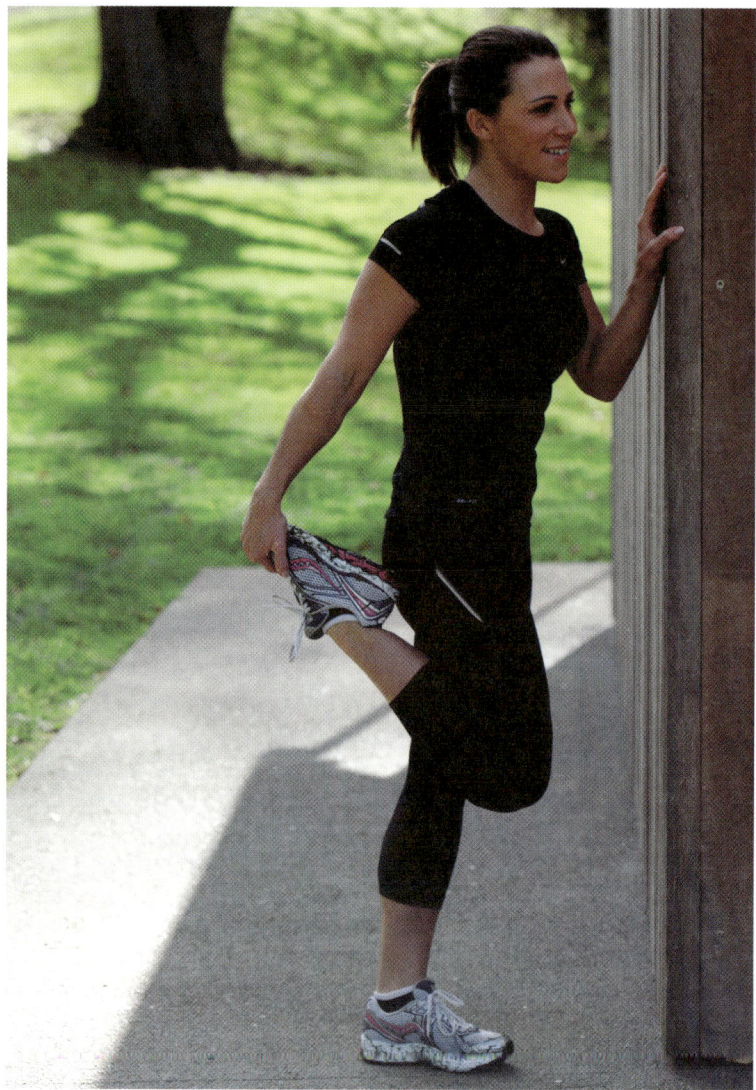

months to increase the time you are physically active as well as increasing the intensity. The biggest thing is to do something every day and that you get into a routine with your fitness and also mix it up to keep things interesting.

Much like your food, you need a plan. It may be that you plan to start walking every morning before work for half an hour and, over time, build some of these walks into runs, add some stretching and maybe a few weight classes or sessions at the gym. Or it could be that you join a netball team and then get some friends together to go swimming a few times a week. It is all about starting somewhere, making it a regular thing and making sure it happens.

What will you do?

It's time to make a commitment to yourself. What are you going to do to get yourself more fit?

Even if you are active now, look at what you can do to up your game. Can you extend your walks? Add some interval training? Start doing some weights at the gym? Want to do a mini-triathlon? Do the Tongariro Crossing? Cycle the Otago Central Rail Trail?

Close your eyes and think about what you would love to be able to do.

YOU TIME: Short-term fitness goal

What would you like to achieve in the next few weeks?

_____
_____
_____
_____
_____
_____
_____

YOU TIME: Medium-term fitness goal

What would you like to achieve in the next few months?

_____
_____
_____
_____
_____
_____
_____

YOU TIME: Long-term fitness goal

What would you like to achieve in 12 months' time?

_____
_____
_____
_____
_____
_____
_____

Overcoming excuses and barriers

In the same way that there never seems to be a good time to start a healthy eating regimen, there is never going to be a perfect time to start exercising if you don't already. Today is as good a time as any. There will always be a list of reasons why it is too hard and excuses to hide behind. Maybe it's because you have got a big project on at work, or deadlines to meet or the kids take up all your time – but that's life. Even if you don't think you can make changes, you *can* – you have choices. If you were told it was a 100 per cent life or death situation, that you would die tomorrow at 8 a.m. if you didn't start exercising, I can guarantee that most people would be able to stop wasting time on something, shuffle their day around a bit and just make things work to fit in that 30 minutes a day – if your life depended on it. I know what you might be thinking, that right now it's not life and death for me – but in some way, it really is.

If you are currently very unfit, it can be extremely overwhelming to start being more active: often it hurts, you may feel irritated that you can't walk or run as far as you used to and you may have a list of excuses which you use to justify why you can't get moving. The truth is, though, you can get over all of those things – if you choose to. It is all about starting somewhere and building on that.

If you have always hated exercise and never been fit at all, you can still do something to change this and you are never too old to begin. If you are always comparing yourself with a fitter you 10 years ago before you had children, or you are angry at yourself for letting your fitness slide, these negative thoughts will get you nowhere. It is time to forgive yourself for anything from the past, accept 100 per cent responsibility for yourself right here, right now and choose to make a change – that's my challenge to you.

It is a really good idea to think now of all the excuses you use, all the reasons why it may be too hard to exercise or all the barriers that you might come across and find some solutions. Here are some examples:

Excuse	Solution
I don't have time!	Look at your diary, identifying at least three 30-minute time slots where, if you moved things slightly, you would be able to at least do something towards getting fit. Monitor your daily activities for one week.
	Make exercise a part of your daily routine. Maybe walk or cycle to work. Walk to the shops, take the dog for a longer walk, take your trainers to work and go for a walk at lunchtime. Whoever you are, there will be something you can do.
	Always take the stairs when you can.
My friends and family don't exercise.	It doesn't necessarily mean they won't; talk to everyone you know and see if there is someone who would be keen to walk, run or go to gym classes with you.

Excuse	Solution
Lack of energy and motivation.	Work out what time of the day you are most energetic and plan to exercise then.
	See if you can exercise with other people by joining a sports club or group exercise class.
I travel a lot.	Fear not, so do I! It doesn't mean that you can't be active. My exercise gear is the first thing I pack when I head away, anywhere. Pack a skipping rope in your suitcase.
	Wherever you are, you can walk or run. Look online to see if there is a swimming pool or gym near to where you are staying and build some time into your schedule for exercise. Communicate this to the other people you are travelling with, if necessary, so they know what your plans are when you arrive at your destination.
I have injuries.	I know how hard and frustrating it can be when you want to exercise but certain injuries make it difficult. Most of the time, though, there will be SOMETHING you can do. Seek the advice of a qualified fitness professional to help you come up with a plan.
I can't afford to join the gym.	Walking, running, skipping, squats, press-ups, sit-ups and similar exercises don't have to be done at the gym. Check out the exercise plans on page 120 onwards for tips on how to exercise without needing equipment.
It is raining and cold outside.	You can actually exercise in the rain you know! That's what raincoats and umbrellas are for. Alternatively, find something else to do. Have a plan for things you can do if the weather turns against you: indoor cycling, swimming, stair climbing, skipping, dancing or gym work.
I have a busy family life and no time!	Exercise with your kids. Walk together, play running games or tag. There are also fitness computer games you can do as a whole family.
	Trade babysitting time with a friend, neighbour or family member who also has small children. Offer to look after their kids for an hour so they can have some time out, and they can then return the favour and you can get active in this time.
	Exercise when the kids aren't around or when they are sleeping – there are lots of things you can do in your own home.

YOU TIME: What's holding you back, and what's the solution?

So, let's look at your problems and barriers and think up some solutions which might work for you – don't skip this, it is IMPORTANT! We are about DOING, remember. Let's get some results! Either draw yourself a blank table on a separate piece of paper, or alternatively write into the gaps below. First, I want you to think of all the problems and barriers in your life that are preventing you from exercising. Then alongside each problem, write in your solution.

Excuse	Solution

Sample exercise plans to get you started

Over the next few pages you will see some sample exercise plans to help get you started on your exercise regimen. Below are some detailed descriptions of some of the individual exercises to help you learn how to perform these correctly.

Squats

- Stand with your feet slightly wider than hip-width apart, keep your chest lifted and your chin parallel to the ground.
- Engage your abdominal/core muscles (in other words, keep your tummy tucked in!).
- Bend at the knees and lower your hips until your thighs are almost parallel to the ground (just like sitting on a chair). Make sure your knees don't go over your toes as you squat down.
- Push through your heels and squeeze your bottom to return to a standing position.

Adapt it: to make it more challenging, try holding weights or milk bottles filled with water in each hand.

Push-ups

- Move to a hands-and-knees position on the floor with your hands directly under your shoulders, fingers facing forward.
- Reach one leg out and away and then the other leg to come into a plank position so your hands and feet are supporting your whole body weight.
- Engage your abdominal/core muscles.
- Bend the elbows and slowly lower your body towards the floor until your arms bend at right angles. Keep your back straight and abdominals tight.
- Press upwards through the arms and push yourself away from the floor – again keep your back straight.

Beginners: to make this exercise easier, you can keep your knees on the ground.

Lunges

- Stand with your feet hip-width apart and engage your abdominal/core muscles.

- Keeping your left foot on the ground, step forward with your right leg and lower yourself into a lunge – how far you lunge will vary from person to person. If you are a beginner, just go as far down as feels comfortable; if you are more experienced you should be able to lunge down until your right knee nearly touches the ground.
- Firmly push off with the right leg and squeeze both your thighs and bottom muscles to allow you to return to the standing position.
- Repeat on the opposite leg.

Adapt it: to make it more challenging, try holding weights or milk bottles filled with water in each hand.

Triceps dips

- Sit on the edge of a low bench or stable chair and position your hands shoulder-width apart on each side of your hips.
- Keeping your hands on the bench/chair, move your bottom in front of the bench/chair. Keep your legs slightly bent and your feet hip-width apart on the floor.
- Slowly bend your elbows and lower your upper body until your upper arms are nearly horizontal to the floor – be sure to keep your back close to the bench.
- Once you reach the bottom of your triceps dip, slowly press off with your hands and push yourself back to the starting position.

Adapt it: to make it more challenging you can place your feet on another chair or low bench.

Step-ups

- Find a stable bench that is level with your knee – either at the gym, or find a step somewhere in your house or at the park.
- Stand in front of the bench/step with your knees hip-width apart.
- Step up onto the bench/step with your right leg allowing your left leg to lift off the ground.
- Stand on top of the bench/step with both feet and step back down leading with the right leg followed by the left leg.

Adapt it: to make it more challenging, try holding weights or milk bottles filled with water in each hand.

Front plank (also known as Bridge or Hover)

- Lie on your front on the floor with your elbows close to your sides and directly under your shoulders, palms down and fingers facing forward.
- Engage your abdominal/core muscles.
- Contract your thigh muscles, straighten your legs and flex your ankles (tuck your toes towards your shins).
- Lift your torso and thighs off the floor, making sure that your shoulders are directly over your elbows.
- Hold this position for as long as you can, keeping your back straight and tummy in tight the whole time, then allow yourself to relax and repeat.

Beginners: to make this exercise easier, you can keep your knees on the ground.

Side holds

- Lie on your right side on the floor with your knees slightly bent and legs stacked on top of one another. Engage your abdominal/core muscles.
- Keeping your hips and bottom in contact with the floor, raise your torso and support yourself on your right forearm. Your right elbow should be bent and directly under your shoulder.
- Lift your hips and bottom off the floor until your shoulder, hip and knee are in a straight line. Keep your tummy tight and hold this position for as long as you can. Relax and then repeat on the other side.

Note: to make this more challenging you can lift your lower leg off the ground, too.

For more information about individual exercises, head to my website, www.claireturnbull.co.nz.

Now it's time to look at some sample exercise plans. Each one of the following plans has been customised to suit your current level of fitness (whether you are a beginner, intermediate or advanced) and whether or not you have gym access.

Beginner with no gym access

If you do little to no exercise right now, this is a good place to start.

Day	Activity
Monday	30 minutes cardiovascular exercise at an easy to moderate intensity. Try a mix of walking, jogging, bike riding or swimming.
Tuesday	10 minutes brisk walking + 20 minutes resistance training. Do 15–20 repetitions of each of the exercises below, then repeat them all another 2 times through so you are doing 3 sets in total. • Squats • Push-ups • Lunges • Triceps dips • Front plank.
Wednesday	REST DAY
Thursday	30 minutes cardiovascular exercise at an easy to moderate intensity. Try a mix of walking, jogging, bike riding or swimming.
Friday	10 minutes brisk walking + 20 minutes resistance training. Do 15–20 repetitions of each of the exercises below, then repeat them all another 2 times through so you are doing 3 sets in total. • Squats • Push-ups • Lunges • Triceps dips • Front plank.
Saturday	30 minutes cardiovascular exercise at an easy to moderate intensity. Try a mix of walking, jogging, bike riding or swimming.
Sunday	REST DAY

Beginner with gym access

If you go to a gym, here are some alternative exercises you could do.

Day	Activity
Monday	30 minutes cardiovascular exercise at an easy to moderate intensity. Try a mix of treadmill, cross-trainer, rowing machine or bike.
Tuesday	10 minutes cardiovascular exercise + 20 minutes resistance training. Do 10–15 repetitions of each of the following exercises, then repeat them all another 2 times through so you are doing 3 sets in total.

Day	Activity
Tuesday *continued*	• Leg press • Seated row machine • Dumbbell squats • Chest press machine • Front plank.
Wednesday	REST DAY
Thursday	30 minutes cardiovascular exercise at an easy to moderate intensity. Try a mix of treadmill, cross-trainer, rowing machine or bike.
Friday	10 minutes cardiovascular exercise + 20 minutes resistance training. Do 10–15 repetitions of each of the exercises below, then repeat them all another 2 times through so you are doing 3 sets in total. • Leg press • Seated row machine • Dumbbell squats • Chest press machine • Front plank.
Saturday	30 minutes cardiovascular exercise at an easy to moderate intensity. Try a mix of treadmill, cross-trainer, rowing machine or bike.
Sunday	REST DAY

Note: ask a trainer at the gym to help find the right weight for you and to explain how to use the machines correctly – it is really important that you are exercising safely.

Intermediate with no gym access

Either progress to this after a month or two on the beginner's programme or start here if you already have a basic level of fitness.

Day	Activity
Monday	45 minutes cardiovascular exercise at a moderate intensity. Try a mix of walking, jogging, bike riding or swimming.
Tuesday	15 minutes brisk walking/running + 30 minutes resistance training. Do 10–15 repetitions of each of the exercises below, then repeat them all another 2 times through so you are doing 3 sets in total. • Squats (try holding weights/bottles of water in each hand as you squat) • Push-ups • Lunges (put front leg on a step to add intensity) • Triceps dips (put your feet on a box to add intensity)

Table continues overleaf

Day	Activity
Tuesday *continued*	• Step-ups (find a step at least 30 cm high and aim for a controlled movement). • Front plank • Side holds.
Wednesday	45 minutes cardiovascular exercise at a moderate intensity. Try a mix of walking, jogging, bike riding or swimming.
Thursday	15 minutes brisk walking/running + 30 minutes resistance training. Do 10–15 repetitions of each of the exercises below, then repeat them all another 2 times through so you are doing 3 sets in total (see Tuesday notes for intensity). • Squats • Push-ups • Lunges • Triceps dips • Step-ups • Front plank • Side holds.
Friday	45 minutes cardiovascular exercise at a moderate intensity. Try a mix of walking, jogging, bike riding or swimming.
Saturday	15 minutes brisk walking/running + 30 minutes resistance training. Do 10–15 repetitions of each of the exercises below, then repeat them all another 2 times through so you are doing 3 sets in total (see Tuesday notes for intensity). • Squats • Push-ups • Lunges • Triceps dips • Step-ups • Front plank • Side holds.
Sunday	REST DAY

Intermediate with gym access

Either progress to this after a month or two on the beginner's programme or start here if you already have a basic level of fitness.

Day	Activity
Monday	45 minutes cardiovascular exercise at a moderate intensity. Try a mix of treadmill, cross-trainer, rowing machine or bike.

Day	Activity
Tuesday	15 minutes cardiovascular exercise + 30 minutes resistance training. Do 10–15 repetitions of each of the following exercises, then repeat them all another 2 times through so you are doing 3 sets in total. • Dumbbell squats • Lat pulldown machine • Dumbbell lunges • Dumbbell chest press • Leg curl machine • Front plank • Knee tucks.
Wednesday	45 minutes cardiovascular exercise at a moderate intensity. Try a mix of treadmill, cross-trainer, rowing machine or bike.
Thursday	15 minutes cardiovascular exercise + 30 minutes resistance training. Do 10–15 repetitions of each of the exercises below, then repeat them all another 2 times through so you are doing 3 sets in total. • Dumbbell squats • Lat pulldown machine • Dumbbell lunges • Dumbbell chest press • Leg curl machine • Front plank • Knee tucks.
Friday	45 minutes cardiovascular exercise at a moderate intensity. Try a mix of treadmill, cross-trainer, rowing machine or bike.
Saturday	15 minutes cardiovascular exercise + 30 minutes resistance training. Do 10–15 repetitions of each of the exercises below, then repeat them all another 2 times through so you are doing 3 sets in total. • Dumbbell squats • Lat pulldown machine • Dumbbell lunges • Dumbbell chest press • Leg curl machine • Front plank • Knee tucks.
Sunday	REST DAY

Note: Ask a trainer at the gym to help find the right weight for you and to explain how to use the machines correctly.

Intermediate/advanced with no gym access

For those of you who have a really good base fitness, this level of training might be more suitable!

Day	Activity
Monday	60 minutes cardiovascular exercise at a moderate intensity. Try a mix of walking, jogging, bike riding or swimming.
Tuesday	15 minutes brisk walking/running + 45 minutes resistance training. Start experimenting with the exercises you have been doing (look back at those in the intermediate section), try changing the order of exercises, number of sets and repetitions you do. Also you can start to add more resistance using ropes, small logs, larger plastic water containers . . . be creative!
Wednesday	45 minutes high-intensity interval training (mix up what you do – running, bike, etc). Try 1–2 minutes high-intensity cardiovascular exercise followed by 30–60 seconds recovery.
Thursday	60 minutes cardiovascular exercise at a moderate intensity. Try a mix of walking, jogging, bike riding or swimming.
Friday	15 minutes brisk walking/running + 45 minutes resistance training. Start experimenting with the exercises you have been doing (look back at those in the intermediate section). Try changing the order of exercises, number of sets and repetitions you do. Also you can start to add more resistance using ropes, small logs, larger plastic water containers . . . be creative!
Saturday	45 minutes high-intensity interval training (mix up what you do – running, bike, etc). Try 1–2 minutes high-intensity cardiovascular exercise followed by 30–60 seconds recovery.
Sunday	REST DAY

Intermediate/advanced with gym access

For those of you who have a really good base fitness, this level of training might be more suitable!

Day	Activity
Monday	60 minutes cardiovascular exercise at a moderate intensity. Try a mix of treadmill, cross-trainer, rowing machine or bike.

Day	Activity
Tuesday	15 minutes cardiovascular exercise + 45 minutes resistance training. Talk to your gym instructor about changing your programme by adding new exercises, more resistance, changing the tempo you exercise at. Don't be afraid to ask; your gym instructors are there to help!
Wednesday	45 minutes high-intensity interval training (include boxing or indoor cycling classes). Try 1–2 minutes high-intensity cardiovascular exercise followed by 30–60 seconds recovery.
Thursday	60 minutes cardiovascular exercise at a moderate intensity. Try a mix of treadmill, cross-trainer, rowing machine or bike
Friday	15 minutes cardiovascular exercise + 45 minutes resistance training. Talk to your gym instructor about changing your programmes by adding new exercises, more resistance, changing the tempo you exercise at.
Saturday	45 minutes high-intensity interval training (include boxing or indoor cycling classes). Try 1–2 minutes of high-intensity cardiovascular exercise followed by 30–60 seconds recovery.
Sunday	REST DAY

Thanks to Dave Margison at www.workout.co.nz for his support with these plans.

SLEEP

I have had the great fortune of working alongside Dr Alex Bartle for the last few years who, after 30 years working as a GP in a private practice, now focuses on helping people with sleep problems. From working with Alex and talking to people about sleep for the last few years, I have learnt so much. Sleep is just the most fascinating thing and a totally overlooked part of health and wellbeing, if you ask me. It is absolutely as important as what you eat and how much you exercise. So, be sure to read on . . .

Why is sleep so important?

Sleep is your body's time to rest and recover, and without good-quality sleep everything in life can seem much harder. When you have inadequate good-quality sleep (I emphasise the quality), it is hard to think, concentrate and generally function on a day-to-day basis and, in short, you are cheating your-self if you don't get enough. Most people need around seven hours' sleep a night, but this really does vary from person to person. The reason I talk about the quality of sleep is that simply being in bed with your eyes closed for seven hours isn't enough; you need to make sure that you are doing the right things to help your body go through the phases that it needs to so you are getting the best from your kip.

If you aren't sleeping well right now, it is likely to be something you need to look at to help you on your weight-loss journey and to move towards better health and wellbeing. Some people think there is nothing that can be done to help you sleep well, but there absolutely is if you are talking to the right people. No one should have to live without good sleep – it makes you nutty!

What happens when you sleep?

When your head hits the pillow you might not think much is happening between the time your eyes close and the time you wake up – but you couldn't be more mistaken. Sleep is a very active process and at times your brain is as active at night as it is during the day.

When you are sleeping, you go through what are known as sleep cycles. Basically, over a period of around 90 minutes, you will go from light sleep into deep sleep and then up into a lighter sleep again. At the top of the phase (in light sleep) you often wake up, roll around or move, but unless you have someone snoring next to you, or you have one of those massive alarm clocks with huge red numbers glaring in your eyes, you are likely not to remember having woken up at all.

Both phases of sleep are very important and have different functions.

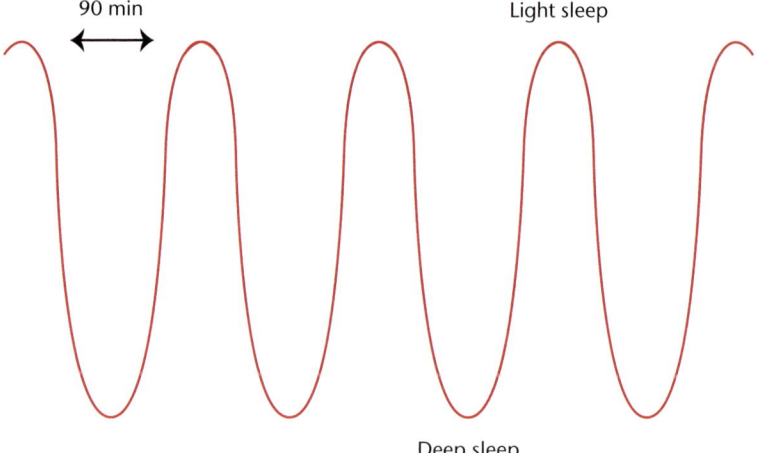

90 min

Light sleep

Deep sleep

Light sleep or rapid eye movement (REM) sleep

REM sleep is a very important lighter phase of sleep, although its exact function is not fully understood. Important brain chemicals become inactive and are allowed to accumulate. When we wake, we then have an abundance of these chemicals available that help with our emotional wellbeing and awareness. They seem to prepare us for waking. You are most likely to have dreams during REM sleep.

Deep sleep or non rapid eye movement (NREM) sleep

Deep NREM sleep is when your body is in physically restorative mode, and helps you to feel re-energised and rested upon wakening. Inadequate deep sleep can leave you feeling fatigued and groggy.

What affects the quality of your sleep?

People delight in telling me that they can have a coffee just before bed and they sleep just fine. Take a deep breath: you are about to hear some bad news. Having caffeine in your system when you go to sleep won't necessarily stop you going to sleep or stop you from staying asleep, but it will stop you going into your DEEP sleep. What this means is that even though you may sleep for seven, eight or nine hours, the quality of your sleep will have been poor; because stimulants have been hanging around in your body, it couldn't go into the deep restful sleep that it needs to allow you to wake up feeling rested. So what happens? Well, you wake up and probably need a coffee to get you going, and so the cycle throughout the day continues. This is where my passionate HATE for energy drinks comes into play, especially when children are drinking them. On top of our ever-growing coffee culture, adding these caffeinated energy drinks with a combination of stimulants into the mix is just creating havoc in my opinion.

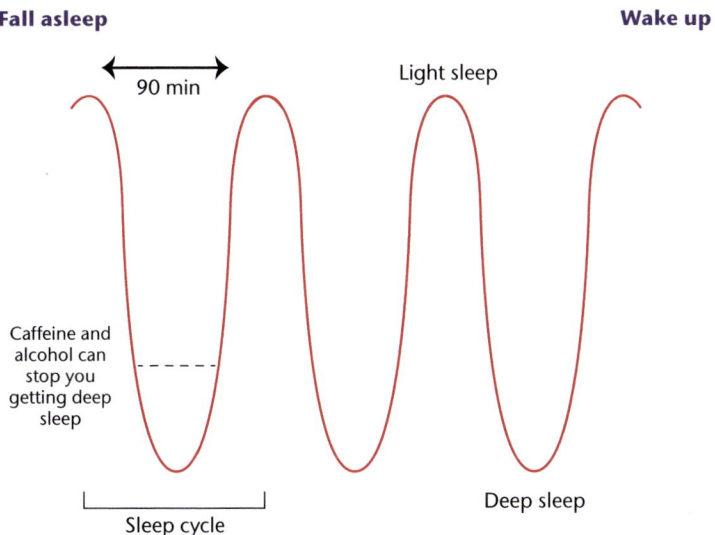

Note: this is a very simple pictorial description of sleep cycles. In truth they are much more complex. Speak to Dr Alex if you want to know more (www.sleepwell clinic.co.nz).

So my advice is to limit your coffee or tea to one or two a day and keep them to the earlier part of the day. If you are a highly stressed person, anxious or sensitive to caffeine, I would suggest cutting it out altogether.

Alcohol has a similar effect to caffeine – you might feel like it knocks you out and helps you to sleep, but the broken-down products of alcohol also stop you from going into deep sleep. Another reason not to drink too much.

Sleep and your weight

There is more and more evidence that inadequate sleep can affect your weight. Your body produces hormones (leptin and ghrelin) which play an important part in regulating your appetite. When you have inadequate sleep, the regulation of these hormones can be affected and as a result, how much you want to eat is also affected. In other words, tiredness leads to you feeling hungry. In addition, when you are tired from lack of adequate sleep, motivation to do exercise is likely to be reduced.

Healthy sleeping habits

✓ Aim to get around 7–8 hours' sleep each night.
✓ Try to go to bed and get up at the same time each day – this helps keep your body clock synchronised.
✓ Get outside in natural daylight every day – this helps your body to produce melatonin which is one of the hormones that regulates sleep cycles.
✓ Get regular exercise every day – this can help you sleep better. Try not to do intensive exercise too close to bedtime, as this can keep you awake.
✓ Bed is for sleeping – avoid watching TV in bed or doing work in bed.
✓ Make your bedroom comfortable. It's important that your pillow, mattress and bedding are all comfortable – you spend a lot of your life sleeping, and sleeping well is essential.
✓ If you wake up constantly during the night and become anxious, get out of bed, keep warm, try to relax by reading and return to bed after about 20 minutes; it will help you sleep. Also, when in bed, don't look at the clock. It will only stress you out if you know that you have to get up in a few hours.
✓ Allow yourself time to wind down before bed.
✓ Balance what you drink – too much fluid and you will need the loo during the night; not enough, you can wake up thirsty.
✓ Avoid large, heavy meals at night and try to leave an hour or so between your meal and sleeping.

If you need help with your sleep, give Alex a call, he is brilliant! You can also visit his website for more information: www.sleepwellclinic.co.nz.

So now you have the knowledge you need about nutrition and digestion, have a good idea of what you need to be eating and drinking to help your body work at its best, know the ins and the outs of weight loss, know what exercise you need to be aiming to include, as well as a good understanding about the importance of good-quality sleep. But as you know, Lose Weight for Life is not just about what you know, but how to APPLY what you know to get the outcome you want. Read on . . .

3

Making Things Happen

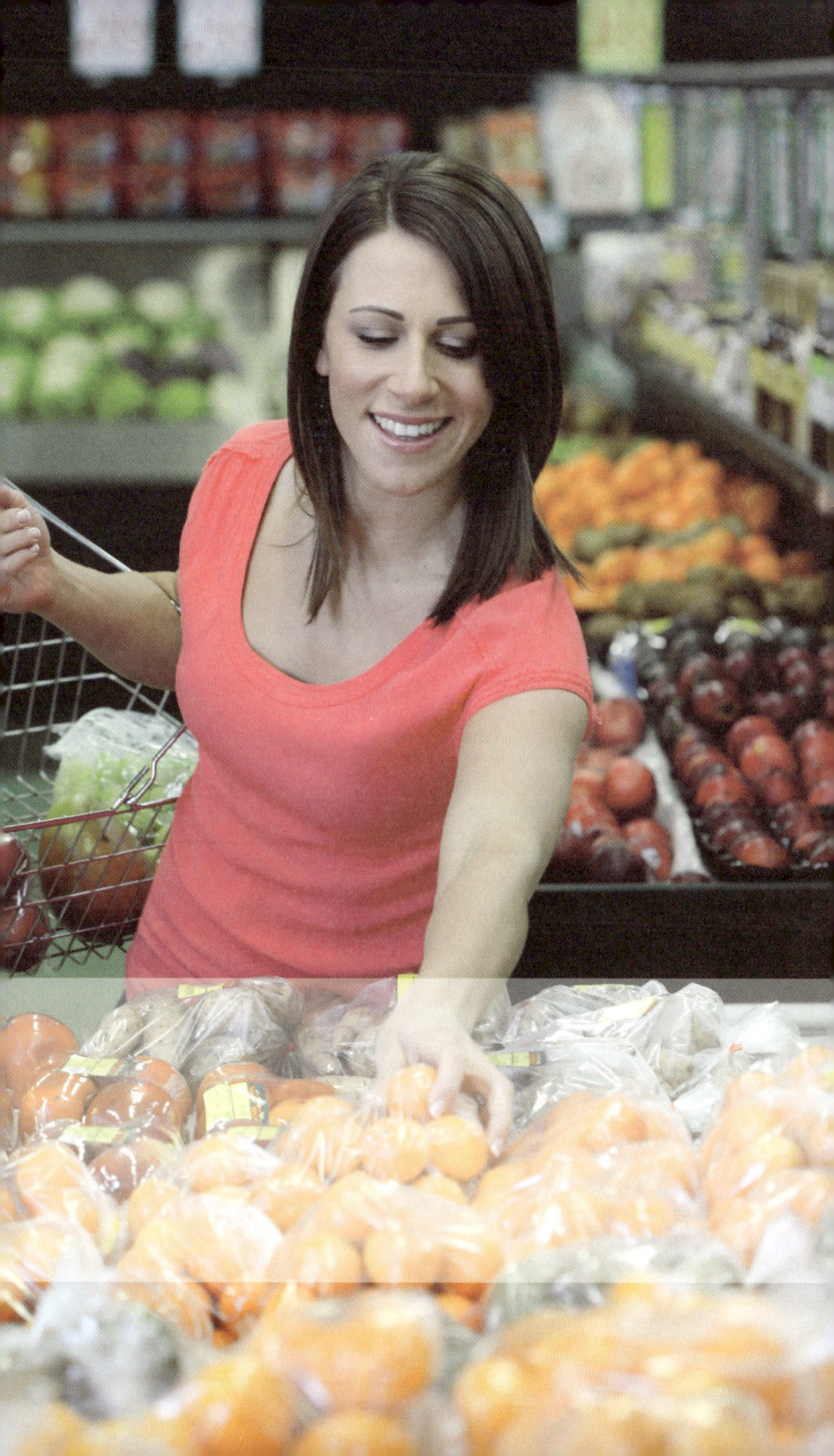

So far we have looked at who you are and where you want to be as well as focusing on the way you eat and where you need to start changing things. You have set a vision and identified some goals to work on – hurray!

We have cleared up the confusion when it comes to nutrition, food, exercise and wellbeing. I hope you have a good idea of what foods you need to be eating each day to help your body work at its best and feel totally and utterly fantastic. But now comes the really exciting part, the part where we make the magic happen!

Information, ideas and theory aren't enough to get you where you want to go or to get you the results you deserve. It is time to apply everything you have learnt so far to your life.

There will be many things to work on in this coming section, so remember, it is not about trying to change all these things overnight; this is a process, a JOURNEY to a beautiful and fabulous destination.

Look at all these areas and do ONE thing at a time. When you have addressed that, and it is ingrained into your being, move on to the next. This process may take a few months and that is totally fine; good things will come and it is so worth it – and far better than a quick fix which ends up with you right back where you started. So, let's focus. Your time to shine is now . . .

To help guide you through this next section, below is a summary of the main topics we will be covering:

Part 1: Creating habits and routines that stick

HOW DO I KNOW WHAT TO EAT EACH DAY?

One of the most challenging things about eating well is pulling together everything you know about healthy eating into some kind of plan so you actually know what to eat for breakfast, lunch and dinner.

The easy way out is to download a meal plan from the internet or to follow one from a weight-loss article in a magazine – but this isn't ideal. These plans won't be personalised to you, they often aren't easily adapted and the sheer fact that someone else has done it for you takes away the skills you need to learn to do this for yourself. I know, I know . . . the easy way will seem far more appealing, BUT – I promise you – if you want to Lose Weight for Life, you need to do things for yourself. This will allow you to form new habits and behaviours and to make changes that last!

So, how can you easily put together a fabulous eating plan by yourself?

Solution: build yourself a plan

Let's recap on what you need to be aiming to include in a whole day:

Fruit	2 servings a day*
Non-starchy vegetables	3+ servings a day*
Starchy foods	Small amounts at each meal, preferably foods which have been minimally processed
Dairy products, including milk, yoghurt and cheese	2–3 servings a day*
Lean meat, poultry, fish, seafood, eggs and legumes	1–2 servings a day*
Fats and oils	Small amounts of healthy fats
Water	Plenty!

*A serving is roughly what fits into the palm of your hand.

To build yourself a healthy meal plan, you need to work out combinations of meals and snacks which allow you to get the right balance of foods over a whole day. Some of you might like to have the same structure each day, for example at breakfast always having 1 serving of fruit, 1 dairy serve and something starchy. Others of you will no doubt like to mix it up. Do whatever works for you.

There is no need to over-focus on the plan (again, please don't forget the bigger picture – it's what you eat most of the time that makes the biggest difference), but use your plan as a rough guide to make sure that on most days you are getting the balance you need.

There will be instances when you won't have a whole serving at one time; for example, you may have a little grated cheese in a sandwich which is only half a serving. You can just have the other half serving at another time during the day, but you don't need to get too bogged down with this. Start by trying to get a basic structure together and accept that there will be small variations on a day-to-day basis.

In the following pages are some healthy meal plans for people I have worked with based on around 6000 kJ a day – these guys were all trying to lose weight. Have a look at them and then try to put together your own plan. You can write as many meal plans as you like, and then use these to help you sort out your weekly meal planner and shopping list on pages 140–1. Note: data for healthy meal plans was gathered using Foodworks 2009.

Diane is in her late thirties, loves food and everything about eating. She works from home and prefers to have a more substantial breakfast after exercising in the morning and a lighter dinner at night. Here is how we made things work for her.

Meal time	Meals	Food group
Breakfast	• Porridge with ½ cup of oats and 1 cup of low fat milk with 1 small apple, grated • 2 brazil nuts (for selenium) Alternatives: you can make porridge with quinoa or brown rice to which you can add berries or dried fruit instead	• Healthy starch • Fruit • Dairy products **kJ = 1400**
Lunch	2 large handfuls of salad (lettuce, spinach, capsicum, bean sprouts, cucumber, beetroot, tomato) with ¾ cup of leftover roasted kumara and pumpkin with 100 g of chicken and a few nuts	• Non-starchy veggies • Healthy starch • Lean meat • Healthy fats **kJ = 1750**
Dinner	120 g of salmon with 2 cups of stir-fried red onion, broccoli, cauliflower and carrots with ½ cup of cooked brown rice (optional) – use garlic and a small amount of reduced-salt soy sauce and chilli to flavour the veggies	• Fish • Veggies • Healthy starch (if needed) • Healthy fats **kJ = 2600**
Snacks	• 1 pottle of low-fat yoghurt • 1 pear or other fruit	• Dairy products • Fruit **kJ = 520**
Hydration	Water and herbal teas throughout the day, maximum of 1 instant coffee or a long black with a splash of milk or a cup of tea	
Total	• 2 servings of fruit • 3+ servings of non-starchy veggies • Starchy foods at most meals • 2 servings of dairy products • 2 servings of lean meat/fish • Small amount of fat • Water! **kJ = 6270**	

Notes about this plan:
- When including dairy products, lower-fat options are best.
- Put your favourite oil into a spray pump bottle which will allow you to use less and keep the kilojoules down.
- Measure your portions of the starchy carbs you have to ensure you are serving yourself an appropriate amount.
- LOTS of non-starchy veggies are used here, with variety being the key.

Tony is in his forties, has a very busy job which requires him to be on the road most days and at the moment he currently eats on the run. He needs quick and easy things to eat in the daytime which he can pack the night before (made while he is prepping dinner), and likes to feel full after eating.

Meal time	Meal	Food group
Breakfast	Smoothie with ½ cup of berries, ½ cup of low-fat milk and ½ cup of water, ½ cup of unsweetened yoghurt, 1 tbsp of oats, 1 tsp of honey and 1 tsp of ground LSA (linseed, sunflower seed and almond mix). Add a splash of chilled water to thin the smoothie down if needed and ice to make it cold!	• Fruit • Dairy products • Healthy starch • Healthy fat **kJ = 800**
Lunch	• Sandwich with 2 slices of wholegrain bread with salad, 100 g of tuna, 1 slice of avocado used as a spread and extra grated carrot • 1 pottle of low-fat yoghurt and a small banana	• Healthy starch • Fish • Non-starchy veggies • Healthy fat • Dairy products • Fruit **kJ = 2050**
Dinner	150 g steak with 1 cup of roasted (in 1 tsp of oil) kumara, potato and carrots with 2 cups of mixed green vegetables	• Lean meat • Healthy starch • Healthy fat • Non-starchy veggies **kJ = 2160**
Snacks	• 1 large raw carrot • 10 mixed nuts • ¾ cup of dried Mini-Wheats (cereal) to munch on	• Non-starchy veggies • Healthy fat • Healthy starch **kJ = 1030**
Hydration	Water and herbal teas throughout the day	
Total	• 2 servings of fruit • 3+ servings of non-starchy veggies • Healthy starch at each meal • 2 servings of dairy products • 2 servings of lean meat/fish • Small amount of fat • Water! **kJ = 6040**	

Notes about Tony's plan:
- When including dairy products, lower-fat options are best.
- Put your favourite oil into a spray pump bottle which will allow you to use less and keep the kilojoules down.
- Check the weight of your meat portion before cooking it.
- Use veggies as snacks!

Sara is 28, doesn't eat meat or fish, but does have eggs and dairy products. She loves cooking! She is keen on eating everything home-cooked if possible and likes smaller meals and filling snacks. She is a late riser and goes to bed late, so likes a good-sized evening meal. She also wants to still be able to enjoy a little bit of chocolate.

Meal time	Meal	Food group
Breakfast	• ½ cup of unsweetened low-fat yoghurt with ½ cup of stewed apple (or rhubarb) and 2 heaped tbsp of home-made muesli which includes nuts and seeds • 2 brazil nuts	• Dairy products • Fruit • Healthy starch • Healthy fat **kJ = 930**
Lunch	• 1 cup of mixed salad greens, 1 small tomato with 1 cup of chickpeas, 2 tbsp of peanuts with a good squeeze of lemon juice as a dressing • Glass of low-fat milk or 1 pottle of low-fat yoghurt	• Non-starchy veggies • Protein alternative • Healthy fat • Dairy products • Fluid **kJ = 1250** Note: chickpeas have some starch too
Dinner	• 150 g tofu and 2 cups of stir-fried (in 1 tsp of sesame oil) veggies, with 2 tsp of sesame seeds and ½ cup of cooked brown rice • 1 orange for after	• Protein alternative • Non-starchy veggies • Healthy fat • Healthy starch • Fruit **kJ = 2420**
Snacks	• 1 small carrot, 1 stick of celery and ½ a capsicum chopped up with 3 tbsp of hummus • 1 boiled egg • 1 pottle of low-fat yoghurt • 2 squares of dark chocolate (high-percentage cocoa)	• Non-starchy veggie • Protein (from egg and hummus) • Dairy products **kJ = 1450**

Sara's plan continues overleaf

Meal time	Meal	Food group
Hydration	Green tea, water, lemon and water	
Total	• 2 servings of fruit • 3+ servings of non-starchy veggies • 3 servings of dairy products • Healthy starch at each meal • 3 servings of protein alternatives • Small amount of fat • Water! **kJ = 6050**	

Notes about this plan:
- When including dairy products, lower-fat options are best.
- Hard-boiled eggs can make a great snack.
- Low-fat yoghurt is a great base for a healthy breakfast.
- To aid the absorption of non-haem iron from non-meat sources, have a piece of fruit which is high in vitamin C as part of the same meal.

YOU TIME: Make your own meal plan

The starting point is to reflect on how much you need to eat in a day, and how you will divide this food up between meals and snacks. As a recap, look back to the table on page 134 to see what is a good guide for most adults of what you need to be eating each and every day to get the balance of nutrients to help your body function at its best and still lose weight. Then, try to fill in the blank meal plan below. If you prefer, you can copy the plan into your own notebook and make more than one.

Meal time	Meal	Food group
Breakfast		
Lunch		
Dinner		
Snacks		

Meal time	Meal	Food group
Hydration		
Total	__ servings of fruit __ servings of non-starchy veggies __ servings of dairy products __ healthy starch at most meals __ servings of lean meat/fish or protein alternatives __ small amount of fat __ water!	

Note: the number of times to eat in a day will vary from person to person and the portion sizes will depend on your current weight and weight-loss goal. For a person-alised meal plan, to work out exactly how many kilojoules you need, what vitamins and minerals you may be falling short on and how to pull this all together, come and see us at Mission Nutrition (www.missionnutrition.co.nz).

HOW DO I MAKE SURE I EAT WHAT I NEED TO?

You can know everything there is to know about good nutrition and what you SHOULD be eating, but if you get home late from work after a nightmare day, have 110 things to do that evening and don't have a plan for dinner that night, regardless of your best healthy living intentions, takeaways, toast or biscuits for dinner will be looking like the appealing option.

Solution: plan meals and make a good shopping list

I totally understand that the words 'meal planning' may fill you with dread, but I can honestly say taking 5–10 minutes a week to write a rough plan of what you will be eating and putting a quick shopping list together will save you so much time (and money) in the long run. It is something I do religiously, WITHOUT fail, wherever I am, because it works. It allows you to apply 'what you know' to 'what you do' in a very painless and easy way and it has GOT to be better than wandering aimlessly around the supermarket at the end of the day, when you are tired (and hungry), trying to work out what to buy for dinner. I don't know how people do that!

So, time to get the equipment you'll need together:

- 1 piece of A4 paper
- 1 pen
- Your desire to eat better and be healthier!

So far, so good! Okay, here goes . . .

Step-by-step guide to POWER planning:

Step 1: Fold your piece of A4 paper in half.

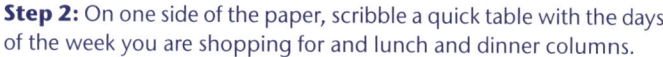

Step 2: On one side of the paper, scribble a quick table with the days of the week you are shopping for and lunch and dinner columns.

Step 3: On the other side, put the name of your supermarket and then butcher and fruit and veg shop if you buy those things elsewhere.

Step 4: Starting with dinners, decide what you would like to eat that week. Think NOW about when you are going out, what you have got on, etc. I would look at having red meat 1–2 times, chicken 1–2 times, fish 1–2 times and some kind of vegetarian or egg-based meal about once a week (I always have an omelette on my busiest night).

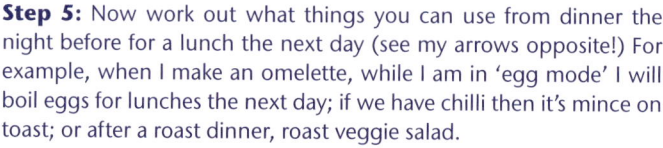

Step 5: Now work out what things you can use from dinner the night before for a lunch the next day (see my arrows opposite!) For example, when I make an omelette, while I am in 'egg mode' I will boil eggs for lunches the next day; if we have chilli then it's mince on toast; or after a roast dinner, roast veggie salad.

Step 6: On the day when leftovers won't make anything for lunch, what else can you have? Soup? Salad? Frittata? Sandwiches? Jot it down, so you know what you are having.

Step 7: Write your shopping list on the side of the page that has the places you shop. Start with what you need for dinners, then lunch and then think about the basics: cereal, milk, yoghurt, snacks, etc.

Step 8: Now add the non-food items you may need: washing-up liquid, paper towels, etc.

Step 9: Shopping time.

Step 10: Pop the plan on the fridge so everyone knows what you are having. You may end up with two or three things in each box if you are catering for a few different lunches.

	Lunch	Dinner
SUN	Sandwiches and fruit	Roast chicken, roasted veggies and green veg ++
MON	Roast veggies / chicken salad	Chilli with rice and salad
TUE	Leftover chilli	Fish and salad (with chickpeas)
WED	Salad with tuna	Veggie/lentil curry and rice
THUR	Left-over curry	Omelette with salad
FRI	Mixed salad with egg	Salmon couscous with spinach
SAT	Leftovers	SHOP TIME!

SUPERMARKET

milk	couscous
yoghurt	bread – wholegrain
nuts/seeds	canned tomatoes x 2
eggs	balsamic vinegar
cottage cheese	green tea
tuna	oats
kidney beans	crackers
chickpeas	frozen peas
lentils	frozen berries
rice	paper towels
olives	washing-up liquid

MEAT/FISH

chicken to roast
mince (500 g)
fish – white (4 fillets)
salmon (500 g)

FRUIT/VEG

fruit (variety)
veggies to roast
 (pumpkin, carrot,
 kumara)
onions, sprouts, spinach,
broccoli, cabbage, lettuce,
cucumber, tomatoes,
avocado

Note: This is an example of a shopping list and assumes that you already have some basic food items in the pantry at home.

Doing this has saved me SO much money and encourages me to try new things. Every week, I will try to make one new recipe to keep things interesting.

Now, you don't have to eat things in the particular order you have written them down; there may be days when, for whatever reason, the meal you planned won't work or you just don't fancy it. No worries, you can mix it up. If you go out for dinner one night that wasn't on your plan and you end up with the ingredients for a meal that you didn't eat, just put it into next week's menu planner.

YOU TIME: Is planning your meals something you need to work on? If so, tick here ☐

What do you need to do to put this plan into action?

_____
_____
_____
_____
_____
_____
_____
_____
_____
_____
_____
_____
_____
_____
_____
_____
_____
_____
_____
_____

BACK-UP MEALS

If your life is anything like mine, there will be days when things go completely pear-shaped and no amount of forward planning could have predicted what ends up happening. In these cases, after a rotten day, if you don't feel like cooking it is a great time to have a back-up meal available. This should be something you can throw together in an instant that is still good for you and not going to sabotage your weight-loss goals.

Solution: back-up meal ideas

Here are some of my go-to meals for when the day has got away on me:

- Frozen fish fillets with oven chips and frozen peas.
- Poached eggs on a slice or two of grainy toast (bread can be from the freezer) with spinach, tomato and/or mushrooms depending on what you have in the fridge.
- Baked beans on grainy toast.
- Soups (make extra and freeze some for times like this), with grainy bread or crackers and some cottage cheese.
- Fresh filled pasta (e.g. tortellini) with some frozen veggies.

YOU TIME: Is having back-up meals available something you need to work on? If so, tick here ☐

What do you need to do to put this plan into action?

_____
_____
_____
_____
_____
_____
_____
_____
_____
_____
_____
_____
_____
_____
_____
_____
_____
_____

WHAT DO I BUY WHEN I AM SHOPPING?

For many people, the supermarket is an overwhelming and confusing place and no sooner do you pass through the one-way cattle-style gates than you want to run out screaming – particularly if it is really busy and everyone seems to have trolley rage going on.

If you know what you are going in to get (yay for shopping lists!) and feel like you have the knowledge and skills to interpret the food labels and to confidently make the best choice within each food category, then voilà, stress levels decline and the experience will be a lot more enjoyable. To be honest, when you get back to eating good-quality whole foods such as fruits and veggies, whole grains, unsweetened low-fat dairy, lean meat or fish, eggs, nuts and seeds and healthy fats, shopping becomes quite straightforward and you don't end up having to read that many labels. So that's a good long-term goal.

But for now, based on where you are today, here are my helpful hints to make your food shopping problems disappear forever.

How do I read a food label?

Reading food labels can be a NIGHTMARE. It can be impossible to work out what they are trying to tell you – so let's start from the beginning.

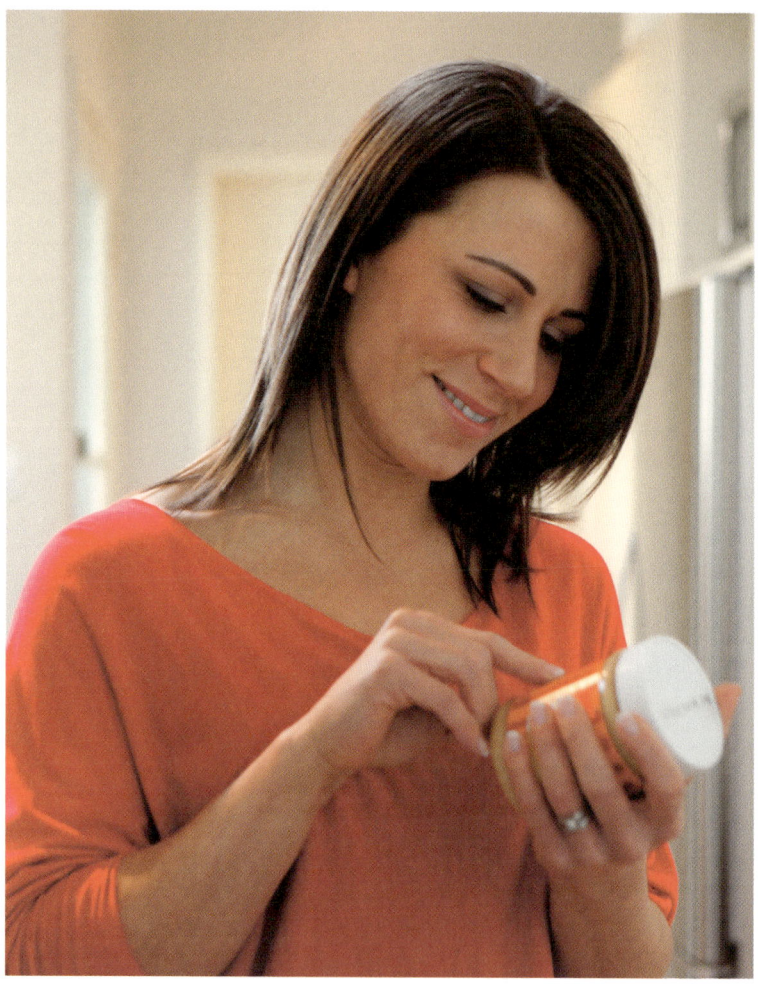

What is on a food label?
- Name or description of the food
- Ingredients list
- Nutrition information panel
- Storage and cooking instructions
- Date mark: use by and/or best before date
- Allergen warnings.

What does the information on the nutrition information panel mean?
The nutrition information panel has a breakdown of all the different nutrients which are in the food. At the minimum this panel must state the energy (kJ), protein, total fat, saturated fat, carbohydrate, sugar and sodium. When claims

are made about the food product (e.g. when a claim is made about the type of fat in a product) more detail will be required; with fat as an example, the amount of monounsaturated and polyunsaturated fat would also need to be listed.

Here is an example of a nutrition information panel on a bread product:

Nutrition information: bread Servings per package: 8.5 (15 slices & 2 crusts) Average serving size: 88 g (2 slices)			
Content	**Avg qty per serving**	**% DI* per serve**	**Avg qty per 100 g**
Energy	800 kJ	9%	910 kJ
Protein	7.9 g	16%	9.0 g
Fat, total – Saturated	0.9 g 0.2 g	1% 1%	1.0 g 0.3 g
Carbohydrate – Sugars	35.6 g 2.8 g	11% 3%	40.4 g 3.2 g
Dietary fibre	3.6 g	12%	4.1 g
Sodium	375 mg	16%	425 mg

Ingredients: Water, Wheat Flour, Mixed Grains (24%), (Wheat, Rye), Skim Milk Powder, Wheat Gluten, Iodised Salt, Vinegar, Yeast.

* Percentage daily intakes (DI) are based on an average adult diet of 8700 kJ. Your daily intakes may be higher or lower depending on your energy needs.

As we discussed on page 60, bread is a carbohydrate-rich food – i.e. a high proportion of it is carbohydrate – BUT it does have small amounts of other nutrients such as protein, fat and fibre as well as vitamins and minerals.

The 'per 100 g' column of a food label will tell you how much of each of these nutrients is in 100 g of that specific food. So in this bread, per 100 g, there is 9 g of protein, 1 g of fat (of which 0.3 g is saturated), 40.4 g of carbohydrate (of which 3.2 g is sugar) and there is 425 mg of sodium. You will also see that fibre is listed, with this bread having 4.1 g. Fibre doesn't legally have to be listed on a food product, but often is on products with a decent amount of fibre to make sure you know that product is packed with something good!

What do the 'per serving' columns mean?

Food manufacturers commonly suggest a serving size for their food product, for example 2 slices of bread, ¾ cup of cereal, 2 Weet-Bix or 150 g of yoghurt may be 1 serve. These are not standardised, though, and do vary from product to product. The numbers under the columns here indicate the amount of each nutrient that is in the given serve as specified by the food manufacturer.

From a weight-loss point of view, though, don't assume that the serving is the right amount for you to be eating; it is only a starting guide.

What does the '% of DI' mean

On some foods there is a column which says how much of a percentage of your recommended daily intake (DI) or dietary allowance (RDA) the nutrient is.

What this means is how much of a particular carb, protein, fat, fibre, vitamin or mineral this food has, based on the average 8700 kJ person's needs for different nutrients. For example, with the bread product, 2 slices provides 9 per cent of total energy needs for the day, 1 per cent of fat and so on.

HOW DO I MAKE THE RIGHT FOOD CHOICES WHEN I AM TRYING TO LOSE WEIGHT?

It really comes down to two things: making the best choice in each food group and eating the right serving size for your needs.

1. Making the best choice in each food group

When you are looking at a food product and its nutrition information, you are looking at different things depending on what you are buying. For example, with savoury products such as crackers, the key things to compare would be fat, saturated fat, fibre and sodium. With peanut butter (which is always going to be a high-fat food because it's made with nuts), the things you are looking for are the highest percentage of nuts and the least added sugar and fat – and preferably New Zealand made.

Different foods have different rules. Within each food category (let's take crackers, for example), there is unlikely to be one variety which is the absolute stand-out, best one. There will probably be two or three varieties that are similar-ish: one may be slightly lower in fat but higher in sugar, the other may have a tad more sugar but less sodium. It would be impossible to pick an absolute winner. Overall, therefore, with most food categories, you are looking for the best few options within the range.

If you reflect back to your goal about what you need to be eating in a day, let's see what you would be looking for within each of these categories.

Food group	Category	What to look for
Fruit		With fresh fruit, the fresher the better. Frozen fruit can be fantastic – berries, for example, are brilliant in smoothies or on porridge. If you do use canned fruit, go for one packed in juice rather than syrup.
Vegetables		As with fruit, the fresher the better – try to grow your own or buy from a local supplier or farmers' market where you know the produce is fresh. Frozen vegetables are a great back-up option, and most have nothing added to them; just check the ingredients list to be sure.

Food group	Category	What to look for
Starchy foods	Starchy vegetables	This group includes potatoes, kumara, yams, green bananas, taro and corn. When purchased fresh, none of these will come with a nutritional information panel, so the key thing here is portion size. Use no more than a small fist-sized amount at a meal.
	Rice	Provided you are looking at plain rice, there is no need to look at the numbers on the nutritional panel. Go for brown rice, ideally, and if you use white rice go for basmati as it has a lower GI than other white rice – this means it is more slowly absorbed by your body. Portion size is key – don't cook more than you need.
	Pasta	As with rice, dried pasta is dried pasta and brands will be very similar nutritionally. Wholemeal pasta is higher in fibre. Overall, the amount you cook and eat is the most important thing to consider.
	Breads	Dense wholegrain breads with lots of fibre are your best bet. Go for the option with the highest amount of grains, not just one with the odd grain here and there. Choose a thin-sliced option where possible.
	Crackers	Wholegrain crackers are ideal everyday crackers. Look for those with: • Less than 5 g fat/100 g and less than 1 g saturated fat • More than 5 g fibre/100 g • Less than 500 mg sodium/100 g where possible. Rice crackers and corn crackers are lower in fibre and won't fill you up as much (and can be high in sodium), but are a good choice when you are entertaining and far better than potato chips.
	Breakfast cereals	Good old oats are the way to go. If you are buying plain oats with no flavours added, the numbers on the panel will all be the same. The amount you cook is the thing to remember. I also use quinoa and brown rice as a breakfast base sometimes.

Table continues overleaf

Food group	Category	What to look for
Starchy foods *continued*	Breakfast cereals *continued*	With muesli or other breakfast cereals, the things to look for are how much sugar, fat and fibre it has. Ideally, go for a cereal with: • Less than 10 g fat/100 g and as low in saturated fat as possible • Less than 15 g sugar/100 g (up to 25 g if lots of dried fruit) • More than 7 g fibre/100 g. How much cereal you have is important, too. Even if it meets these criteria, if you have 2 cups it will be far too much for most people who are watching their waistline.
Dairy products	Milk	• Trim milks (including calcium-enriched varieties) have less than 0.2 g/100 ml of fat and are ideal for most adults, particularly those watching their weight. If you use an alternative milk for any reason (soy or rice, for example), try to make sure it is also less than 0.2 g fat/100 ml. • Low-fat and full-fat milks are around 1.5% and 3.3% fat respectively. This might not sound much, but when you drink several 100 ml glasses of milk at a time, it adds up: a cup of full-fat milk has 10 g of fat in it, 2 tsp worth of butter. Not to be sniffed at.
	Yoghurt	• Unsweetened, low-fat, live natural yoghurts are best and absolutely my first choice. Less than 1 g/100 g fat is a good starting point. This can be fresh or packet make-your-own yoghurts. • If you are on a weight-loss mission and looking for a fruit yoghurt, either add fruit to the unsweetened one (ideal) or look for a lite version that is under 400 kJ a pottle.
	Cheese	• Cottage cheese, reduced-fat ricotta and extra-lite cream cheese can be good everyday choices. • With hard cheeses, it comes down to the amount you use. Edam is 25% fat (a quarter of the block), whereas mild, colby and tasty are over 30% fat (a third of the block). Overall, less is best and grate or only use thin slices when you are watching your waistline.

Food group	Category	What to look for
Lean meat, fish and protein alternatives	Meat	• With fresh meat, you are looking for the leaner cuts. With mince, premium is around 5% fat, prime 10% fat and choice 15% fat. • Sausages can be like little fat-sponges so aren't ideal to have too often. They can also be high in sodium. If you do occasionally have them, go for ones with less than 10 g /100 g fat (less than 5 g would be even better), and ladies you probably only need one, men, maybe one or two – not three plus . . .
	Fish	Variety is your best bet and have it as often as you can. Try to have New Zealand king salmon at least once a week. If buying canned fish, look for those in spring water.
	Eggs	The best quality you can afford – I always choose free-range.
	Pulses	• Lentils, chickpeas, kidney beans. If you compare brands of any of these items when they are dried, you will find that they will be nutritionally very similar, so buy what best suits your budget. Where possible, cook pulses yourself. • If you do buy canned varieties, be sure to drain and rinse them and consider how much you eat of them.
	Tofu	Go for plain varieties and season it yourself with garlic, chilli, ginger and reduced-salt soy sauce or any other combination of healthy flavours.
Healthy fats	Oils	My top choice is a good-quality extra virgin olive oil. Other options are ricebran and canola oil. Use oil from a spray bottle if you can so you use less, because all oil is high in kilojoules. For salads, I like flaxseed oil.
	Spreads	• If you choose to use a spread, go for a good-quality one based on the healthy oils. Lite versions are whipped with water to give them fewer kilojoules per serving. • Only use small amounts. • The Heart Foundation tick can be a helpful guide when looking at spreads. • Alternatively, try using avocado, hummus or nut butters as a spread.

Again, the good news is if you are eating lots of real, whole foods, you won't end up having to look at too many labels anyway – that makes life easier. We teach people about label reading and making the best food choices on super-market tours at my nutrition clinic, Mission Nutrition. If you want to know more, come along to one of these!

YOU TIME: Is making the right food choices something you need to work on? If so, tick here ☐

What do you need to do to make this plan happen?

_____
_____
_____
_____
_____
_____
_____
_____
_____
_____

2. Eating the right serving size for your needs

Once you have selected the best product from the range available, the next thing to consider is how much you need. See below for guidance on portions.

WHAT PORTION SIZE IS RIGHT FOR ME?

These days it can be pretty tricky to work out what a normal or healthy portion size is. Go to one café and they might give you a bowl of soup that is barely 150 ml, in another place you might be overwhelmed by a monster bowl which looks like it could feed a family. Same goes for sandwiches: a 'portion' can go from a small sandwich made from two thin slices of bread to a foot-long beast or something that resembles a doorstop more than a light lunch.

Overall, there are a lot of people who are eating too much, and that goes for those choosing the 'healthy option', too. Even if you get the wholemeal grainy sandwich with lean meat and salad, if you need two hands to hold it, it is likely to be more than your body needs.

If we look at the serving sizes of food from 100 years ago we would be shocked and horrified at the difference between then and now. We are led to believe that more is better value for money and bigger is better – but, really, you are simply paying for extra food to make you fat. And, in the long run, that is absolutely NOT cheaper, is it? Think of all the running, gym classes and nutritional advice you would need to help shift that 'free upsize' or coffee and muffin combo that is ONLY $5! There is NO such thing as free when it comes to loading extra kilojoules.

Based on a 6000 kJ day, if you were having three meals and two snacks, this is roughly how you could divide up your kilojoules:

Meals	Snacks
1600 kJ each (with breakfast probably being slightly less and lunch and/or dinner being slightly more)	400–600 kJ each

Keep these figures in mind when looking at the kilojoule content of some of the following foods – you will soon work out which size is right for you.

Breakfast

Now I love a good bowl of cereal as much as the next person, but have you ever looked at the serving size on the packet? In some cases they may seem ridiculously small, but this goes to show that even a healthy food, if you have too much, won't help you lose weight. Here are the kilojoule contents of some natural untoasted mueslis.

Muesli (one which meets the healthy criteria on page 148)	kJ
2 cups	2700 kJ
1 cup	1350 kJ
½ cup	674 kJ
¼ cup	340 kJ

So, considering you are likely to have some milk or yoghurt and fruit with this, the ½ cup portion would be about right for the 6000 kJ day.

Lunch

Sandwiches	kJ/fat
Sandwich made with 2 slices of wholegrain bread, a scrape of hummus, lean meat and salad	1400 kJ, 8 g fat
Large wholemeal roll with chicken, cheese and salad (no butter or dressing)	2800 kJ, 20 g fat
Foot-long meatball sandwich with cheese and mayonnaise	3720 kJ, 30 g fat

Dinner

Cooked dinner (with no added oil/butter/dressings)	kJ/fat
150 g meat with a small potato and salad	1700 kJ, 12 g fat
250 g meat with a large potato and small salad	2800 kJ, 20 g fat
350 g meat with a large potato and small salad	3560 kJ, 26 g fat

Solution: manage your portion sizes

Here are some ideas to help you manage your portions:

- Serve up your veggies or salad first and make sure they cover at least half your plate – this will mean that there is less room for the other stuff.
- Use smaller plates and bowls. It has been shown that you can end up eating more if your crockery is bigger.
- Use measuring cups to get a feel for how much cereal is right for you; also measure your rice, pasta, oats, etc. before cooking or eating them.
- Only buy what you need.
- Do your research – if you eat out a lot, go online and see if you can find nutrition information or some indication of the kilojoule content of what you are buying. You will be very surprised in some cases, I am sure.
- If you do end up buying food from a café, or when you are out and about, if there is too much of it, ask to take the leftovers with you and then have them either for afternoon tea or for lunch the next day.
- Remember it is NOT cheaper in the long run to go for the bigger portion!

WHAT IS THE RIGHT PORTION SIZE WHEN IT COMES TO TREAT FOOD?

I'm sure I won't be the only one to have noticed that muffins these days can be enormous and that you can buy huge cookies which are, in truth, equivalent to nine small cookies (yes, you know the ones I mean). Here is the kilojoule content of some of these treat foods.

Cookies	kJ/fat
Mini cookie (10 g)	190 kJ, 2.5 g fat
Medium cookie (30 g)	575 kJ, 7 g fat
Big cookie (95 g)	1820 kJ, 26 g fat

Muffin – double chocolate	kJ/fat
Mini muffin (30 g)	500 kJ, 5 g fat
Medium muffin (60 g)	1000 kJ, 11 g fat
Mega muffin (160 g)	2650 kJ, 29 g fat
Mega muffin with chocolate topping and ½ flake	3650 kJ, 40 g fat

Milk chocolate	kJ/fat
2 squares from family-sized block (12 g)	270 kJ, 4 g fat
Chocolate bar (50 g)	1115 kJ, 15 g fat
King-size block (85 g)	1896 kJ, 26 g fat
Family-size block (250 g)	5575 kJ, 75 g fat

Solution: get the portion size of snacks right

- Banning these foods all together is not a long-term solution for a lot of people and, certainly for someone who may have an emotional bond with any of these foods, total deprivation may lead to bingeing in a moment of weakness. So, put them into your kilojoule budget – small portions (you can see why from the kilojoule content) a few times a week should be the maximum.
- When you have these treats, sit down without distraction so you can be totally aware of what you are doing and enjoy them.
- If you use any of these foods as an emotional crutch, you really do need to deal with that as a separate issue – more on this later (see page 200).

HOW DO I KNOW HOW MANY TIMES A DAY TO EAT?

There are so many theories about how many times a day you should eat and I have heard them all. Six times a day, every two hours, every four hours, don't eat after 7 p.m., don't eat after 9 p.m. – blimey, does your head hurt as much as mine trying to figure that one out?

The truth is it is important to eat regularly but there isn't a generic one-size-fits-all rule that will work for everyone. We are all different, and when it comes to the timing of our meals and how many times we need to eat in a day, it all depends on who we are, how many hours we are up for, what time we get up and go to bed, and when we do exercise. Let me explain.

Twenty-four hours a day your body is busy working; your heart is beating, your kidneys are busy filtering your blood and your brain is active. Your body is constantly burning fuel. Obviously, though, most of us are not eating every minute of every day (even if we would like to), so what happens is that we end up giving our body the energy and nutrients it needs in a number of meals and snacks throughout the day. When you eat, your body will use some of the fuel from that meal or snack and then some for later, between now and the next time you eat.

During the hours that you are awake, it is helpful to eat regularly to provide your body with a slow and steady supply of fuel which it can use right then and there. If you go hours and hours without eating, go past hungry too often or only eat once or twice a day, you are asking a lot of your body which is trying to supply fuel to your brain, liver, kidneys and other organs, when you haven't really eaten enough. As much as you would like to think that when you ignore your hungry feelings and skip meals your body miraculously burns off all your body fat – sorry, it doesn't. Doing this can be very unhelpful for your metabolism and can also make it difficult for you to shift weight.

Solution: get the timing right

Now this is the highly individualised part. I will use myself as an example and look at a few other people I know to show you how this all works.

I get up at 5.15 a.m. each morning and I go to bed about 9.30 or 10 p.m. Based on this, I eat around five to six times a day; this works for me and is regular enough to supply me with fuel every few hours. My biggest meals are breakfast and lunch with a lighter dinner. This is because I am most active in the earlier part of the day (that is when I exercise and run around a lot), and in the evening I am more sedentary and need less fuel. Ideally, I have my evening meal a few hours before bed, not because it will independently make me fat if I eat it before I sleep, but because it takes several hours to be digested and you don't make it easy for your body when you go to bed on a full stomach. At the weekend, I get up slightly later and go to bed at a similar time, so I get my balance of food in three or four meals plus snacks.

My friend Lisa is a teacher who gets up at 7 a.m. and goes to bed about 9.30 p.m. Based on this, she eats four or five times a day, every few hours. She goes to the gym after school, about 5 p.m. Her afternoon tea is relatively substantial (so she has fuel for training and doesn't pass out with hunger at the gym) and she has a reasonable-sized dinner after the gym to help her recover. Like me, she tries to have her main meal a few hours before bed to allow it time to be digested. Her meals earlier on in the day are lighter as she is less active then.

My brother gets up at about 8 a.m. and goes to bed at 11 p.m. He likes to eat bigger meals and snacks and it works for him to eat around four times a day. He is active all day so he has four medium-sized meals rather than three bigger meals and a snack. That works for him. On days when he exercises during the middle of the day, he will have half of one of his meals an hour or so beforehand and the other half afterwards – so overall, he doesn't eat more on those days and risk gaining weight when he doesn't want to.

See . . . we are all different, THANK heavens! So time to think about your day and what will work for you to get the results you want.

YOU TIME: Do you need to work on the timing of your meals? If so, tick here ☐

What do you need to do to put this plan into action?

_____
_____
_____
_____
_____
_____
_____
_____
_____
_____
_____
_____
_____
_____
_____
_____
_____

HOW DO I COOK HEALTHY MEALS?

Now I love cooking shows on the TV, I love recipe books and I love trying new recipes. But as much as I love the work some chefs do, they can be very heavy-handed with some high-kilojoule, high-fat ingredients. As easy as the dishes they suggest are, many are NOT suitable everyday choices from a nutritional point of view. They are often high on the fat and salt and low on veggies. So, whether you are cooking your own tried-and-tested recipes or ones from a cookbook, here are some things to try to keep it healthy and to help you on your weight-loss journey.

Solution: follow these healthy tips

- Think about the overall balance you are looking for in a healthy evening meal: 2 handfuls of non-starchy veggies per person, a small amount of lean meat or fish or alternative protein and probably some healthy carbs. Adapt your recipes to fit this – it might mean cutting down the meat portion and upping the veggies, or serving a smaller portion of the dish with salad on the side.
- Use oil from a spray bottle or measure out your oil with a teaspoon. Remember, 1 tablespoon of oil is around 500 kJ – the same as 1½ slices of bread.

- A splash of cream in many cases can be substituted with a splash of milk as a healthier option. If a recipe does call for a large amount of cream, a) it is probably not a great thing to be cooking if you are trying to lose weight, b) if you are going to make it, try using a smaller amount of lite cream instead, c) try lite evaporated milk as a substitute.
- A can of coconut cream can be as much as 4000 kJ (yes, you read this correctly, no misprint here!). Based on a weight-loss plan of 6000 kJ per day, you can soon see that using lots of coconut cream is NOT helpful for people trying to lose weight. I know you wouldn't have a whole can, maybe a quarter, but that is still 1000 kJ – as much as a small meal. If you do use coconut cream in cooking, use the lite version or lite coconut milk and use as little as possible; when it comes to eating it, don't cover your plate with the coconut-cream sauce.

WHAT MAKES A HEALTHY SNACK?

Do you find it impossible to know what is healthy to snack on? There are so many pre-prepared snack foods which are either really high in sugar or high in fat, and it can be hard to know what is even good for you out of what is available.

Solution: choose healthy snacks

Let's go back to basics here. A snack in my mind is a mini-meal, an opportunity to get some extra nutrients into your day (some healthy carbs, protein, healthy fat, fibre, vitamins and minerals) and snacks that are packed with sugar and unhealthy fats with no goodness don't cut it. Just because we are surrounded by quick-fix solutions that are the new 'normal' doesn't mean these are what our body needs.

So, for great snacks, which are MUCH more helpful as part of your healthy day, I would suggest:

- A few wholegrain crackers with a scrape of Marmite or Vegemite and cottage cheese; or hummus and tomato; or reduced-fat ricotta and a teaspoon of chutney; or avocado and tomato.
- Sliced banana or apple or pear with some cottage cheese – it's surprisingly good.
- Unsweetened yoghurt with a teaspoon of honey and a tablespoon of muesli stirred into it.
- 8–10 raw mixed nuts and a piece of fresh fruit.
- Home-made unbuttered popcorn.
- A boiled egg.
- Edamame beans.
- Home-made vegetable soup.
- Chopped raw veggies with hummus.

YOU TIME: Is healthy snacking something you need to work on? If so, tick here ☐

What do you need to do to make this plan happen?

_____
_____
_____
_____
_____
_____
_____
_____
_____
_____
_____
_____
_____

HOW CAN I MAKE IT MORE AFFORDABLE TO EAT HEALTHILY?

Let's be honest, these days it isn't always cheap to eat well and when you are looking to lose weight and trying to make sure you are selecting the healthier food options, sometimes it can seem challenging. But fear not, I have some ideas.

Solution: try these affordable ideas

- Always, always, always plan your meals. Have a look at the super-market promotional flyers that come in the post or look online to see what this week's specials are – you can use these to help plan an affordable menu.
- Keep your meat portions down. You really only need 100–150 g per person, so do the maths before you buy meat. Cheaper (but still lean) cuts are still great in stews, casseroles and curries; rump is great on the barbecue rather than more-expensive cuts – just leave it to rest for a few minutes before cutting and slice thinly when you serve it – delicious!
- Go vegetarian a few nights a week. There are some fantastic meals you can make with lentils, chickpeas and kidney beans which are very affordable.
- Add pulses to everything! You can add cooked red lentils to mince dishes to bulk them out and you won't even notice they are there. Add a can of chickpeas, butter beans or any other pulses into a curry, stew or casserole to make your meat go further.

- Frozen veggies are a great alternative to fresh. Just remember to cook them in a small amount of water or steam if you can to retain as much of their goodness as possible.
- Watch your extras: coffee from a café, buying bottled water when you can drink tap and buying lunch instead of taking your lunch to work are all things you can end up spending more money on than you need to.

YOU TIME: Is budgeting something you need to work on? If so, tick here ☐

What do you need to do to make this plan happen?

_____
_____
_____
_____
_____
_____
_____
_____
_____
_____
_____
_____
_____
_____
_____
_____
_____
_____
_____
_____

AM I GETTING ENOUGH IODINE?

Research from the National Nutrition Survey 2009 suggests that most of the adult population of New Zealand is mildly deficient in iodine (a mineral). A huge number of people in New Zealand don't have enough of this mineral. One of the reasons for this is that the soil in New Zealand is low in iodine and it is subsequently not passed up the food chain into what we eat. As a result of this common deficiency, New Zealanders have a re-emerging issue with goitre, which is a swelling of the thyroid gland. This can have an impact on growth and metabolism.

One place where people do get iodine from is iodised salt; unfortunately, though, with the rise in popularity of flaky salts and rock salts (most of which are not iodised), a lot of people have moved away from using standard iodised table salt in cooking. On top of that, the salt which is already in the food we buy (canned food, crackers, biscuits, cereals, etc) isn't iodised – the only food which is required to be made with iodised salt is bread.

With around three-quarters of the salt we eat coming from these processed foods, most of which isn't iodised, on top of a kitchen swap to non-iodised varieties – we have a problem.

Solution: eat more iodine-rich foods

- Buy iodised salt – but no need to be too heavy-handed, we still consume far too much salt overall here in New Zealand.
- Make your own soups rather than relying on canned varieties – if you include salt, make sure it is iodised. Overall, you will make a cheaper soup which is better for you!
- Other sources of iodine include seafood, eggs and seameal custard (made from seaweed). Seaweed itself is also great and I love using nori sheets (the ones used to make sushi). I chop them up and put them in salads or in stir-fries, or bake the strips in the oven with a tiny bit of oil for a snack, or make mini-wraps with them filled with things like salad, sprouts (alfalfa sprouts) and some cooked or raw salmon – yum, yum, yum!

IS MY MEAT TOO FATTY?

Fat on your meat can add to your waistline worries without you realising just how much extra kilojoules it has. Let's say you are aiming for around 6000 kJ a day on your weight-loss journey. Now consider this: if you have 150 g of lean steak completely trimmed with NO fat on the outside, this would be around 950 kJ. Then make this a 150 g steak which still has all the fat around the outside; even though it may not look like a lot, leaving the fat on takes that steak up to nearly 1500 kJ! That is a MASSIVE difference. If you had steak once a week and went from untrimmed to totally trimmed, in one year alone you could lose around a kilo from making this small change!

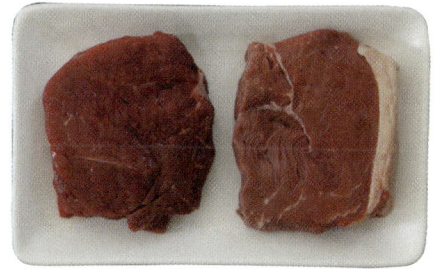

Solution: eat lean

Very simple – if there is any fat on the meat you buy, trim, trim, trim!

YOU TIME: Is eating lean something you need to work on? If so, tick here ☐

What do you need to do to make this plan happen?

_____
_____
_____
_____
_____
_____
_____
_____

WHAT SHOULD I EAT BEFORE AND AFTER EXERCISE?

When you boldly embark on an exercise regimen, it can sometimes mess with the structure of your day. It may be that you can only exercise early in the morning before your day starts, at lunchtime or at the end of the day. Sometimes it can be tricky to work out when to eat. Do you eat a snack before you exercise and your meal after? Or have an early meal and then nothing after? Do you need extra snacks? A minefield, I admit!

Solution: plan your eating around exercise

If you are trying to lose weight, the biggest thing to remember is that you don't want to end up eating more food (i.e. having EXTRA snacks) on top of what you are already eating on a normal day. When you have a handful of extra crackers or an additional serve of fruit and yoghurt, you are just adding extra kilojoules to your day which you are trying ultimately to burn off by doing exercise! So, instead, you need to redistribute the food you would normally eat in a day around your exercise. Here is how it works.

For a morning workout

If you are exercising for an hour or less doing something like a morning walk with the dog, a gym class or cycling which is at a low to moderate intensity, then your body will have enough stored fuel (called glycogen) for you to complete this workout without the need to eat beforehand. Here, though, you just need to eat your breakfast as soon as possible after exercising to help your body refuel and recover. Cereal and milk is fine, but a smoothie made with low-fat milk, yoghurt and fruit is often a great idea after exercise because it gives you a nice dose of carbs and protein to help with recovery.

If you do like to have something in your stomach before a morning exercise session, my advice is to have a small amount of your breakfast before

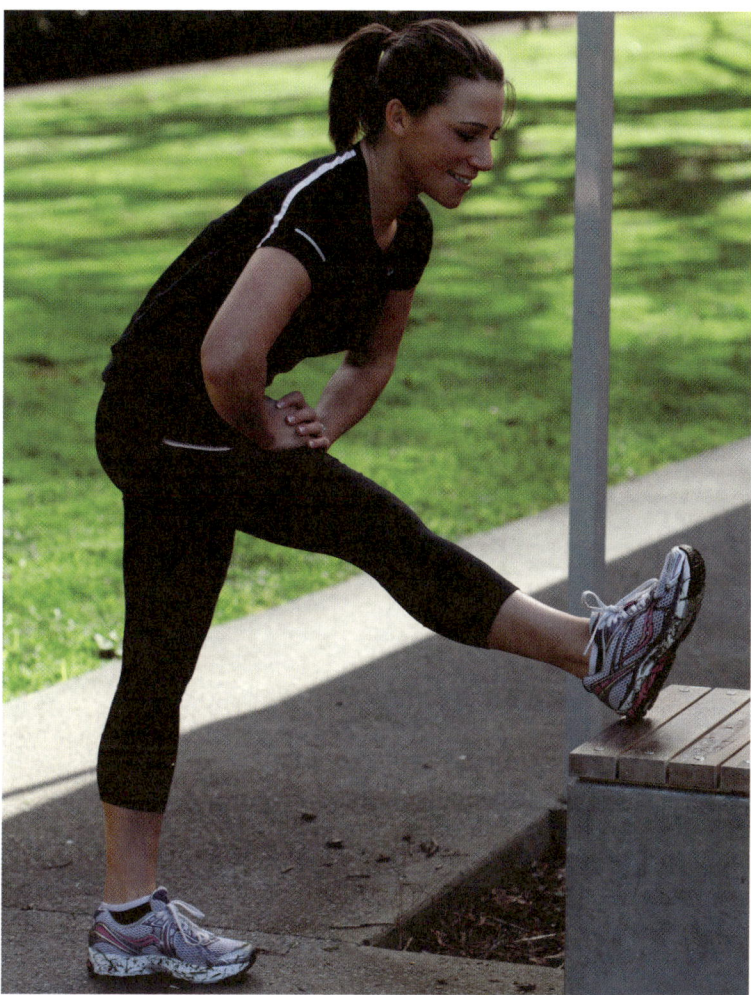

and the rest when you finish. So, let's say you normally have cereal with milk and a small banana; you would have the banana about 30 minutes before you go (to allow it to be digested before you start exercising) and the cereal and milk afterwards.

In both cases you aren't eating more overall.

For lunchtime exercisers

The same applies here; you don't want to add any more food to your day, so, if you normally have a small morning tea (say a piece of fruit) and your lunch is maybe a tuna and salad sandwich with a low-fat yoghurt, I would have your fruit and the yoghurt (from lunch) at morning tea, and then the sandwich after your exercise.

For late-afternoon/evening exercisers

This will all depend on what time you normally have dinner and when you go to bed. If you are heading to a gym class, for a run or for some sport training around 5–7 p.m., I would suggest having a light lunch and a really good afternoon tea like a small bowl of cereal and milk, a sandwich (1 slice of bread) and fruit or a low-fat yoghurt and a banana. Then, after you have finished exercising, have dinner as soon as possible. This may be slightly smaller than normal to make sure you aren't eating more than you need in the day. It is about changing the timing and size of meals rather than adding extras.

If you are exercising later, say 8 or 9 p.m., you might be better to have a small dinner around 6 or 7 p.m. and allow that to digest before you start training. Then have a small snack to assist with recovery when you get back: maybe a glass of low-fat milk, a banana or a low-fat yoghurt.

NOTE: low to moderate intensity means that you finish feeling like you have had a good workout but aren't completely shattered. If you are doing very hard, intensive exercise, you may need additional food and you will also need advice on the exact types of food to be eating before and after exercise to help your body recoup from more intense training. Give us a call at Mission Nutrition if you want to get a plan to help with this (www.missionnutrition.co.nz).

Do you need a sports drink?

One of the key things to remember when it comes to weight loss is the goal of trying to burn off more kilojoules than you are eating each day, thus creating a kilojoule deficit. If you run for one hour you might burn anywhere between 900 and 1500 kJ depending on your weight and how fast you run. A 750 ml bottle of sports drink is over 900 kJ, almost balancing out what you have burnt off. If you are exercising for an hour, water is likely to be adequate afterwards, but remember to have your next meal or snack as soon as possible after finishing to let your body refuel – adding extra kilojoules via a sugar-laden drink is unnecessary.

YOU TIME: Do you need to plan your eating and drinking around exercise? If so, tick here ☐

What do you need to do to make this plan happen?

_____

_____

_____

_____

_____

_____

_____

AM I JUSTIFYING OVEREATING TO MYSELF AFTER EXERCISE?

Have you ever said any of these things to yourself?

- I have been for a run so I deserve an extra glass of wine tonight.
- I worked really hard at the gym this morning, one extra sausage roll won't hurt.
- I walked to get my lunch today so I am sure it's fine to have one of those chocolate caramel slices (2000 kJ a slice when you probably only burnt 40–100 kJ walking to get your lunch!).

I see this justification thing all the time, but it's not helpful! People rarely burn off as many kilojoules in their run/walk/gym sessions as they end up eating with their additional treat food.

Solution: reward yourself with other things

Find other rewards for having worked out hard. Save and buy yourself some new trainers or a new sports top. Avoid using exercise to justify eating more than you need – it can end up being a vicious cycle.

YOU TIME: Do you justify eating treats because you have done exercise? If yes, tick here ☐

What can you do to reward yourself instead of eating?

_____
_____
_____
_____
_____
_____
_____

DO I HAVE A BAD COFFEE HABIT?

Yikes, I know I will be unpopular with some of you for bringing this up, as I am fully aware of how attached some people are to their morning mochaccino or flat white. The thing is, for many of you, a morning coffee and feeling like you NEED a trip to the café for your caffeine fix has become a habit. The same goes for days when you may have meeting after meeting or catch-up after catch-up and end up three or four coffees down by the middle of the afternoon.

Now, there is nothing wrong with the odd coffee, as I have mentioned in Section Two (pages 104–5), but the issue I have here is the habit and routine reliance on it; it's not a good way to go. Coffee made with milk adds kilojoules to your day, for starters. Your average (300 ml) latte made with full-fat milk is 800 kJ; with trim milk it is 540 kJ. If it was one a day, or every other day, that's not so bad. But if coffee is a regular thing, it is highly likely you will be wasting kilojoules that need to be spent on other, good-quality, nutrition-packed foods or just plain low-fat milk minus the coffee!

You may think that swapping to long blacks or black coffee is the answer and, in part, it may be – at least you don't have the kilojoules from the milk. But this raises another issue – the impact of caffeine on your body. While it does indeed act as a nervous stimulant and may, for some, help boost your concentration, your body adapts to caffeine and over time you will need more and more to get the same effect. The other thing, as discussed on page 127, is that caffeine stays in your system for a really long time and can disrupt your sleep.

On top of this, I know MANY people who tell me a coffee is all they have for breakfast and then there are those who routinely end up with a muffin (which, let's be honest, is a cake in a different shape) or some other sweet treat to start off their day – this is not going to help you reach your goal, I promise you.

Don't get me wrong: if you have the odd trim coffee a few times a week and really enjoy it, that might be fine for you. But be truly and deeply honest with yourself, is this a daily habit that needs addressing? A coffee habit could be one of the things leading you away from your goal.

Solution: break your coffee habit

- Rather than heading into the coffee shop in the morning, make yourself a cup of tea (less caffeine and no kilojoules), herbal tea or, even better, have hot water with a few slices of lemon or sprigs of mint. I know, I know – it is not the same as a flat-white fix; but when you make this your normal routine, after a few weeks you will get used to it and wonder how and why you ever used to drink so much coffee. It is just about creating a new 'normal'.
- If you are in meetings, order a pot of English breakfast tea or herbal tea – make it your new 'normal'. You have the power to choose if you want to. If you are in a situation where someone else will automatically buy you a coffee and have it on the table before you arrive, just tell them to order you something else instead. It will only take a few times before they make the change. For goodness' sake, don't drink endless coffee just because that's what everyone else does – that's dumb and not helping you. You are your own person, remember – avoid the trap of doing things just because everyone else is doing it.
- If picking up a coffee is part of your morning routine, change your routine. Drive a different way to work if you need to and, if possible, try to avoid walking past the coffee cart by coming into the office a different way.

- Find something else to help you mentally focus and start the day a better way. Try taking 10 slow deep breaths at some point on your way to work or when you get to your desk. Think about your day ahead and come up with an intention for the day, such as 'be focused', 'be productive' or 'take one thing at a time', write it on a Post-it note and stick it somewhere you can see it. These are the things I do to start my day. You can do what you like, however silly or ridiculous, but find something that helps you start off in a positive way, without needing to rely on a trip to the coffee counter to get into a good head space. A morning coffee is just a habit you have got into and, if you want to, you can change it.

YOU TIME: Is your coffee habit something you need to work on? If so, tick here ☐

What do you need to do to drink less coffee?

_____
_____
_____
_____
_____
_____
_____
_____
_____
_____

DO I EAT TOO MUCH AT DINNERTIME?

When I first moved in with my now husband, I was adapting to buying and cooking the right amount of food to feed both of us for dinner and then have some for leftovers for lunch. The problem was, though, regardless of the amount I cooked, we seemed to end up with very little for leftovers. Does this happen to you?

Here are some of the reasons why this might be happening:

- When you put the food in the middle of the table in 'self-serve' style, while conversation flows and the problems of the world get debated, you may end up picking at the odd extra bit of meat or polishing off another wedge of roasted pumpkin just because it is sitting in front of you – hence, not much gets left for lunch the next day.

- You leave the leftovers on the kitchen bench, or on the stovetop, and you go back for seconds or, worse, end up picking at it while you are clearing up. It can get to the point when you are thinking, 'Well, there is only one tiny bit of meat and one piece of pumpkin left, that's hardly worth taking for lunch, is it? I might as well just eat it.' I know what you're thinking, am I reading your mind?

Either way, you end up eating more than you need to because of habits and behaviours like this. You end up back at square one, with no weight lost!

Solution: eat the right amount at dinnertime

As I have previously mentioned, it takes around 20 minutes after you have eaten for your brain to register that you are full and that you have eaten a meal. In that time, you could have eaten two dinners before you got the 'I am full' message. So, don't leave it to chance; our human minds and wandering forks (or fingers) can lead us to pick at food and eat more than we need.

First, buy and cook the right amount based on the number of people eating and how much you want for leftovers. Buy meat from the butchery counter, or if you buy it in bulk, freeze it in small portioned packs. Measure your rice or other starchy foods before you cook them and only cook what you need. One-third of a cup of dry rice gives you around 1 cup of cooked rice, which is MORE than ample for someone watching their waistline; ¼ cup of dry rice will be more appropriate for most of you I imagine – that is ¾ cup of cooked.

Once you have cooked the right amount, try serving up dinner in the kitchen based on the portion you know is right for you. Only put extra non-starchy vegetables or salad on the table so if anyone picks, they pick at that. When you come to serve up, get out the lunch containers (if you are planning on having the leftovers the next day) and actually serve the 'leftover' portions into these containers at the same time you are serving up the portions for your evening meal – then you shouldn't end up with anything to pick at.

Problem solved!

YOU TIME: Is portion size something you need to work on? If so, tick here ☐

What do you need to do to make this plan happen?

_____

_____

_____

_____

_____

_____

AM I EATING TOO FAST?

Are you one of those people who has already finished your lunch before your colleague has even opened the lid of their lunchbox? If you have ever timed yourself to see how long it takes you to eat a meal or snack, you may be totally horrified. You may think it will take five minutes, maybe 10 – but, I BET you, there will be some of you reading this who can nail a meal in under two minutes and don't really realise how fast you are gobbling your food down. So my challenge to you, tonight or at your next meal, is to time how long it takes you to eat your meal.

So why does it even matter? Well, it takes time for your brain to register that you have eaten, remember.

If you have wolfed down your lunch in three minutes flat, no wonder you may still feel hungry and feel like polishing off a chocolate bar or doughnut. Your poor brain hasn't had time to tell you, 'Excuse me, I have had enough food, thanks.' What can happen is that you eat more than you need to in one go and, also, you can feel overfull before you get the message.

Solution: eat more slowly

Find ways to eat more slowly. Put your fork and knife down between mouthfuls. Aim to chew your food a set number of times before you swallow. Use smaller cutlery so you put less in your mouth at one time. Find something, whatever it is that works for you, to SLOW you down and allow your body the time it needs to register that food has arrived!

YOU TIME: Do you eat too fast? If yes, tick here ☐

What can you do to help yourself eat more slowly?

_____

_____

_____

_____

_____

_____

_____

AM I DRINKING TOO FAST?

You may not realise it, but the size and shape of the glass you drink out of can actually affect the speed at which you drink – it turns out to be a bit of a mind trick. You are more likely to drink slowly out of a tall, slim glass than a short, stubby one.

Solution: pace your drinking

- If you are drinking alcoholic drinks, go for taller, slimmer glasses – it may help slow down your drinking!
- When you are drinking water, go for a wide glass.

YOU TIME: Do you need to pace your drinking? If yes, tick here ☐

What can you do to manage this better?

_____
_____
_____
_____
_____
_____
_____
_____
_____
_____
_____

AM I MINDLESSLY EATING?

You can plan things endlessly when it comes to working out what and when to eat, but there are still things which can trip you up if you are not aware you're doing them. Welcome to the concept of mindless eating.

Mindless eating is when you eat more than you think or make a decision to put food in your mouth without you consciously knowing you are doing it.

Do you ever eat with the TV on? Eat when you are checking Facebook or answering emails? You may end up eating more than you need to, according to the most incredible researcher Brian Wansink who has written a whole book on this topic called *Mindless Eating* (which is well worth a read, by the way).

When you eat while distracted, even if you know everything there is to know about nutrition, your brain isn't really registering the food going into your mouth and you may in part be blissfully unaware of how much you are eating.

If the TV is on at night while you are eating, you are more likely to pick at that extra potato, eat quickly and want seconds before your brain has got a chance to figure out you have already eaten enough.

So, all good intentions and weight-loss hopes and dreams can go out of the window just because you have the TV on when you are having your dinner – it's time to stop this habit and change, change, change!

Solution: eat mindfully

Now there is no need to go overboard, be silent at meal times, worship every mouthful of food and count the number of kilojoules on each forkful. Just be aware. Turn the TV off when you are eating, try not to eat while you are answering emails and take the time to focus on your food, take small mouthfuls, chew properly and be lovingly aware of the delicious things you are eating to nourish your body and mind. It can really make a much more pronounced impact than you realise.

YOU TIME: Are you mindlessly eating? If so, tick here ☐

What can you do to manage this better?

_____
_____
_____
_____
_____
_____
_____
_____
_____
_____

Part 2: Managing hiccups in your daily routine

We are creatures of habit, but some of your small habits, which may go un-noticed, can make a big impact on your ability to lose weight and, of course, keep it off. Here are some really common habits or 'hiccups' in your daily routine which may be having a bigger impact on your weight than you think!

DO I OVEREAT WHEN I AM ENTERTAINING OR BEING ENTERTAINED?

Think back to a time when you have had people round for dinner or a barbecue. You've probably put out an array of different foods: meat, fish, kebabs, potato salad, bread, cheese, crackers, dips and so on . . . (Are you hungry yet?) Anyway, there is a very interesting thing that can happen here.

If you invite people to help themselves, in time your guests will no doubt head to the table and dig into and serve themselves a variety of yummy morsels. Half-full bowls will be left on the table along with the odd sausage or bread roll and a number of other leftover bits. At this point people may have seconds, but while the bowls are all half full your guests may not feel like going back for more food because they can SEE that a lot of food has already been eaten.

What some hosts do (I know I have done this myself) is remove the empty bowls and condense the leftovers onto just a few plates, and leave those on the table as they look much more appealing to your guests. The interesting thing here is that when you do this, it can encourage people to 'dig in' again, because part of their mind has forgotten just how much food has already been wolfed down.

The same goes for the desserts – it somehow seems much easier to have seconds when the big dish of apple crumble you have just devoured has disappeared from the table and now just the ice cream container is left staring at you!

Again, Brian Wansink is the man in the know and has shown very nicely in a study that when students were served chicken wings at a Super Bowl game and were able to order as many as they liked, those who had the remains (the bones) of what they had already eaten removed from sight and were then presented with a clean bowl of chicken wings each time ate around 30 per cent more than those who had the remains left in front of them – that's huge!

Solution: how to eat the right amount when entertaining

The solution here is to be aware that you could be doing this and, in truth, you may even be doing it more than you currently realise. When you go up to a buffet table or serve yourself at a barbecue, try to only go once, look at the food in front of you, serve the green, leafy low-kilojoule salad stuff first (to fill half your plate, remember) and then add some protein and a small amount of something starchy. Then walk away and don't go back. You are unlikely to 'need' extra servings and you will see another meal again! You will be able to have another barbecue and there will be another chance for you to enjoy the foods you love – you don't have to go overboard all in one day.

YOU TIME: Do you overeat when you are entertaining or being entertained? If yes, tick here ☐

What can you do to manage this better?

_____

_____

_____

_____

AM I GETTING CAUGHT OUT WHEN I GO OUT FOR BRUNCH?

When you eat out, you can potentially expose yourself to a whole mountain of unseen kilojoules. One of the times you may least expect this is if you are going out for breakfast or brunch – I mean surely eggs on toast or muesli with yoghurt isn't going to be that high in kilojoules, is it? Well, that all depends – you may be shocked by this . . .

Let's recap. A healthy breakfast based on 6000 kJ a day would be under 1600 kJ and should ideally be providing you with a healthy balance of fabulous nutrients.

Brunch meals

Eggs on toast

Now your standard poached eggs on toast is likely to be the lowest kilojoule option here. Two eggs on two slices of toast without any spreads or butter would be around 1200 kJ and would be a perfectly acceptable 'eat out' breakfast with a cup of tea or hot water.

Where the potential kilojoule overloads come in is with scrambled eggs. These may well be made with a splash of milk and small spray of oil, making them very similar in kilojoules to your poached eggs; but, let's be honest, in a nice café this is highly unlikely. Scrambled eggs are more likely to be 2–3 eggs, cooked in butter and/or oil in an unsparing quantity, and if you want to know

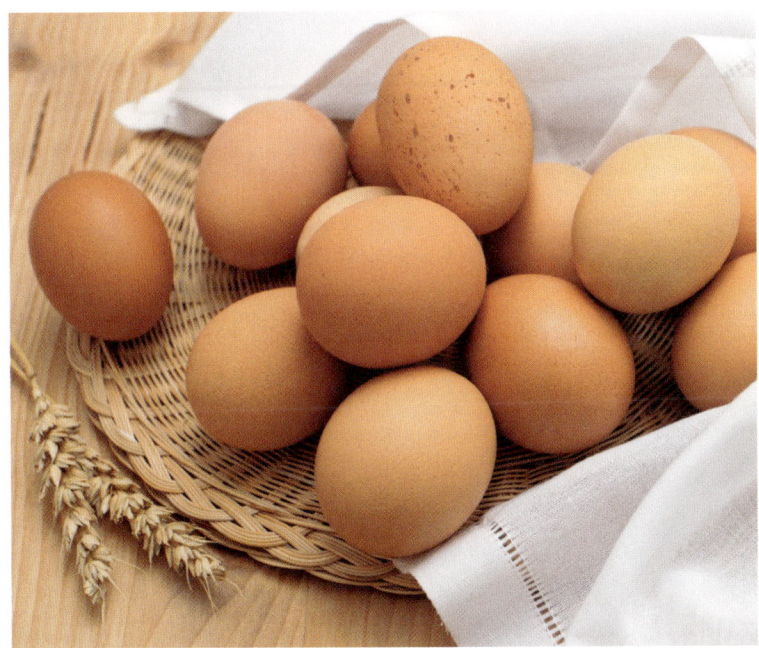

why the eggs look so good on your plate, so light and fluffy, it's often because a splash of cream has been added. This can take your eggs on toast breakfast up to anything from 2000 to 2500 kJ – and that is before you add a side of creamy mushrooms or avocado, and you haven't even ordered a coffee yet!

Eggs Benedict

A true favourite with many, I know. Creamy delicious hollandaise with runny eggs and toast . . . then there is the bacon on the side or, if you prefer, salmon. The hollandaise sauce (2 heaped tablespoons) adds a whopping 1200 kJ to the breakfast; that is nearly as much as the eggs on toast by itself. The four rashers of bacon are an extra 1400 kJ. All up, two poached eggs on toast with hollandaise and bacon and you are looking at spending 3800 kJ from your 6000 kJ of the day. This is also being a little conservative; I have seen nutrition information on café websites with eggs Benedict pulling in at 5500 kJ a serve – yikes!

Cooked breakfast

Well, now you have seen the impact of adding bacon to basic eggs on toast, it will be no surprise that by the time you throw some sausages in there, maybe the odd hash brown and some fried tomatoes, this option is getting up to 4000, 5000, 6000 kJ . . .

Muesli

Reading the numbers above, you may well think that a MUCH safer option is to go for what you think has got to be a good choice: muesli. In many cases you may be right; but you also need to consider that not all mueslis are created equal. Some are made with very little extra fat and sugar and are basically oats with added dried fruit, nuts and seeds. Others are made by coating the oats in a large amount of oil and honey or sugar and then toasting them and later mixing in the fruit, nuts and seeds – these end up kilojoule-wise being comparable to crushed-up biscuits rather than a healthy morning feed.

The next thing to consider is the portion size, which will vary depending on where you go. I have been out for breakfast before and ordered the cereal option and seriously must have been given 1.5–2 cups of the muesli, which may be good value for money but still is FAR more than I need. Even with the healthier type of muesli this would still be 2500–3000 kJ and that is without having added milk, yoghurt or any other extras. I only need about a ½ cup for my weight and size.

Then on to what gets served with the muesli; often in my experience you will get served thick and creamy high-fat natural yoghurt on the side, which with just a couple of tablespoons could add another 500 or more kilojoules to the mix.

Solution: eat well when out for brunch

So, what is the solution? Let's be honest, if you go out for brunch or breakfast only once a fortnight, then staying at home, avoiding your friends and eating your normal breakfast doesn't have to be the answer here. As much as that may help from a weight-control perspective, I am here to help you find long-term solutions to manage your weight in the real world and that includes when you go out and enjoy yourself.

The answer then is to make the best choice you can from the menu – one that is about the right amount of kilojoules as well as providing you with some fabulous nutrition! In most cases poached eggs on wholegrain toast with a side of tomatoes or spinach (if not fried or full of cream) is likely to be the best option. If you get a good look at the muesli and see that it is a healthier-looking one, ask for it to be served with low-fat yoghurt or trim milk if possible, and don't eat it all if you don't need it. Remember it is NOT better value for money to put it in your body when you don't need it – leave it, as hard as that may be to get your head around, it's better in the long run.

Next, consider what you are drinking. I will always go for herbal tea or hot water with breakfast or sometimes normal breakfast tea. I would suggest you do the same where you can.

YOU TIME: Is healthy brunching something you need to work on? If yes, tick here ☐

What do you need to do to put this plan into action?

_____
_____
_____
_____
_____
_____
_____
_____

HOW DO I COPE WHEN I GET HOME FROM WORK AND I'M SUPER STARVING?

Sometimes, after a long day at work or when you have been out and about doing things, you get home and suddenly realise just how hungry you are and feel like you could literally eat anything and everything in sight. Making good food choices at times like this can be near-impossible – so here is what you need to do to manage.

Solution: avoid being super starving

- If this regularly happens to you, change your eating routine slightly. Try having a lighter lunch followed by a decent filling afternoon tea so that when you do get home, you are not out-of-control starving and unable to make a good choice about what to put in your mouth.

Filling afternoon-tea snacks include things like a small bowl of cereal with low-fat milk, fruit and low-fat yoghurt or hummus and wholegrain crackers. I am also a big fan of taking to work a small portion of Bircher muesli (see recipe on page 220) and a low-fat yoghurt if I need something substantial in the afternoon. If you put the muesli into a small plastic container and pack it along with a small tub of yoghurt in a small chilly bag, you can take it with you anywhere.

- If you know you are going to be out and about or very busy at work all afternoon, like a good girl guide you should be prepared. When you leave the house in the morning, grab a banana or make an extra sandwich from one slice of bread for the afternoon.
- If, for whatever reason, you do have biscuits and high-fat and high-sugar foods in the house, keep them in non-transparent containers at the back of the cupboard or pantry so they are not the first thing you see when you open the door.
- Have some chopped veggies such as carrots, celery and capsicum prepped and ready to go right at the front of your fridge. Then, when you walk in from your busy day and open the fridge, these are the only things you see. As well as these standard snacking vegetables, you can also try munching on cherry tomatoes, snow peas and mushrooms if you like them raw (I love them these days!). The best thing to do is to prep these veggies and put them in a container while you are chopping any vegetables for your dinner the night before. If you get into the routine of doing this, it will then become a normal part of your day.
- In winter have a batch of veggie soup in the fridge at all times. You can then head for a cup of that when you walk in to warm you up and fill you up at the same time. The bonus is, of course, more veggies and not too many extra kilojoules.
- Have a LARGE glass of water and/or put on the kettle and make yourself a green or peppermint tea before you think about having something to eat – check that you aren't actually thirsty rather than hungry.

YOU TIME: Do you need to avoid being super starving when you arrive home from work? If yes, tick here ☐

What do you need to do to make this plan happen?

_____
_____
_____
_____

HOW DO I MANAGE WHEN I GET HUNGRY WHILE DRIVING HOME?

There is nothing worse than being starving hungry and having nothing to eat. Blood-sugar levels are low, and you know it will be a while until your next meal . . . the drive-through or the gas station are probably the easiest options but, really, what on earth can you buy from there that's a decent nutritional addition to your day?

I guess you could get a salad from the drive-though – ha ha! – sorry, I am not meaning to be sarcastic but in a moment like that, when you are contemplating eating your arm off, I am doubtful you would give up the fries or burger for lettuce. As for the gas station, it is virtually impossible to find anything healthy in there apart from an overpriced bag of nuts or a less than fresh piece of fruit, if you are lucky. So, if this does sound like you, the best thing to do is to avoid this situation from occurring.

Solution: how to manage your hunger on the way home

- Plan your meals and snacks, first and foremost. If you are out for the morning or afternoon and there is even the remotest possibility that you might end up having to go a long time without food, grab a piece of fruit, or put a washed carrot or a handful of grainy crackers in a resealable food bag. Remember, though, these snacks still need to be counted in the total amount of food you plan to eat that day.
- If you have the ability to keep food in your car without feeling like you have to eat it, it is a good idea to keep an emergency food kit in the boot. This is basically a few food items which you can have if you are going to be home late, or miss a meal because of some drama or something similar. The choices need to be healthier than what you would be picking up from a fast-food place or a gas station.
- Your box needs to be a non-transparent sealed container (so that every time you see it you can't look at the contents and think, um, okay that looks tempting, I will just eat that now). Also, go for things which have a reasonably long shelf-life. You may also need plastic cutlery and food bags to put the rubbish into.
- So, why keep it in the boot? Well, I used to have mine in the glove box and then when I got stuck in traffic, it was all too easy to eat the food when I was just bored and frustrated, not really hungry at all – best to be out of sight and not too easy to access.

My box includes things like:

- Nuts and seeds – SMALL portioned bags
- Tubs of fruit with a spoon
- A liquid breakfast drink

- A tuna and rice pre-mix pot
- Mini tubs of creamed rice
- Small bags of unbuttered popcorn.

YOU TIME: Is eating on the way home something you need to work on? If so, tick here ☐

What do you need to do to make this plan happen?

_____

_____

_____

_____

_____

_____

_____

_____

_____

_____

_____

_____

_____

WHAT SHOULD I DO WHEN MY LUNCH MEETINGS RUN OVER TIME?

Do you always seem to end up in lunch meetings which run over time? Halfway through the meeting your stomach starts growling, you feel a bit faint and you are dreaming about the lunch you have sitting in the fridge which you really wish you had eaten before you came into the meeting. Worse still, by the time you leave the meeting, you have gone 'past hungry' when your body has had to take over and pump some sugar into your bloodstream as you've gone too long without eating. By the time you get to your lunch, you don't enjoy it as much as you thought you would.

Solution: plan your lunch around long meetings

If this sounds like something which happens to you, do what I do. I have half my lunch before and half afterwards. So, say my lunch is a salad with brown rice and chicken, fruit and yoghurt, I would have half the salad with the fruit before the meeting, and the other half with my yoghurt afterwards. Having your blood sugar crash in a meeting is not a good look and can make even the most interesting catch-up painful. Don't let this happen to you; have a plan and be prepared!

YOU TIME: Do you need to have a plan for days when lunch meetings run over time? If yes, tick here ☐

What do you need to do to make this plan happen?

_____

_____

_____

_____

_____

_____

_____

_____

Part 3: Overcoming challenges

Now you have some top tips and ideas about how to establish healthy eating habits and routines, we'll move on to the next part of the Lose Weight for Life programme: overcoming the challenging times. This is the real point of difference in the Lose Weight for Life approach – managing in the REAL world!

Once you are able to identify the challenging times and situations that are holding you back from losing weight and keeping it off, you are then in the driving seat to change things. With the right solutions and strategies, you will be onto a winning streak of results that last, yee ha!

HELP . . . I DON'T HAVE TIME

Life is busier than ever. With technology we are able to check emails at any time of the day on our phones, order food to arrive on our doorsteps without having to go into a shop and book trips away online, but still things don't seem to be getting easier and, unless I am missing something, we still aren't getting a twenty-fifth hour in the day.

It often feels that we are just expected to do more in the time we have saved with these so called 'advances' and it can be impossible to switch off from the busyness of the world. I am sure we have all said a thousand times, 'I would LOVE to do that (sort out the garage, start yoga classes, eat well, etc), but I just don't have enough time.'

The truth is, though, that we all only have 24 hours a day in which to do everything and if you REALLY want to make a change (and you are ready to change, as discussed on pages 36–7, you have to give up using time as an excuse. Accept the reality of your situation and choose to do something differently; no one is going to knock on your door and give you that magic twenty-fifth hour. Harsh, I know, but true.

Solution: do it differently

If you are waiting for the 'perfect' time to start cooking healthier meals, to focus on what you eat and drink or to start being more active, that time will never come. There is no perfect time. The time is now; do one thing differently, build on that and over the course of the coming weeks, months and years, get and maintain the life of health and wellness that you deserve. It is a process and, as Lao-Tzu the famous Chinese philosopher said, 'A journey of a thousand miles begins with a single step.'

YOU TIME: Do you feel like there is never a right time to start eating well? If yes, tick here ☐

What can you do to overcome this and make some changes?

_____
_____
_____
_____
_____
_____
_____
_____
_____
_____
_____
_____

IT IS SO HARD TO EAT WELL AT WORK

Even with the best intentions, with pressing work deadlines, meetings running over time and projects taking longer than you think, it can be tricky to predict your day and, as we know, in life, things change.

I have had conversations with clients in the past who are convinced that it doesn't really matter what they eat at work, provided things are okay-ish at other times – but it does, it really, really does. Think about it: if you are working five days a week, 48 weeks a year, that is 240 lunches and well over 500 snacks each year. If you are having a slightly bigger portion than you need for lunch or making a less-than-ideal choice, then over a year, let me tell you, it counts!

I think some of the biggest challenges when it comes to eating well at work, over and above the busyness and unpredictability side of things, is knowing what on earth to take that tastes nice and can be eaten without too much hassle and mess – oh and, most importantly, doesn't take half an hour to prepare. Fear not . . . I have the answers.

Solution: eat well at work

What to pack for work

The following plan is based on eating lunch, morning and afternoon tea at work and having breakfast and dinner at home. If you are also having breakfast at work, you will need to think about adding my breakfast stash suggestions.

You will need to work out how much of your daily food requirements you have at work. Here is my suggestion:

Food type	Per day	At work (lunch and snacks)
Fruit	2 servings a day	1 serving
Non-starchy veggies	3+ servings a day	1–2+ servings
Starchy foods	Small amounts at most meals	Small amounts at most meals
Dairy, including milk, yoghurt and cheese	2–3 servings a day	1 serving
Lean meat, poultry, fish, seafood, eggs and legumes	1–2 servings a day	1 serving
Fats and oils	Small amounts of healthy fats	Small amounts of healthy fats
Water	Plenty!	Plenty!

So, what can you make from this? Well, if you are having lunch and two snacks at work this is how I would suggest breaking it down:

LUNCH

One to two handfuls of veggies, something starchy and some protein.
Here are some examples:

- Green salad leaves with chopped cucumber, spring onion, cherry tomatoes, leftover cold baby potatoes with a small can of tuna, a hard-boiled egg and a few olives.
- A sandwich made from thinly sliced wholegrain bread, tuna, a slice of avocado and lots of salad.
- A bowl of vegetable and lentil soup, with a slice of wholegrain bread.

In the recipe section of this book I have included some great throw-together lunches which are just fantastic, tasty and far more interesting than just your basic sandwich or salad (see page 228).

SNACKS

One serving of dairy and one serving of fruit. If you have higher energy (kJ) needs, you may need additional fruit or starch, or maybe a second serving of dairy.

Things you could try:

- Wholegrain crackers with cottage cheese and a pear.
- Home-made popcorn, a low-fat yoghurt and an orange.
- A glass of milk and a banana.

BREAKFAST

If you eat breakfast at work, too, you might need a stash of:

- Breakfast cereal (which meets the healthy criteria, see pages 147–8) or ideally some oats to make porridge.
- Tubs of fruit and fresh fruit.
- Low-fat yoghurt and milk.
- Long-life milk for an emergency in case you run out of fresh milk.

So now you know what to eat at work, how can you make sure it happens?

It is all very well having a list of wonderful ideas but, as we have talked about so far, it is just 'theory' until we can make this work for you. Here is how.

You need a plan of how you want to work things with your lunch. I suggest that you either:

- Have a themed week, like a sandwich week, a salad week, a soup week and so on. When you are shopping for food that week, buy things to help you make interesting variations on your theme, so it could be tuna salad Monday, egg salad Tuesday, chicken salad Wednesday and so on. This allows you to vary what you are eating, but makes it nice and easy so that you don't have to think, 'Ah, what on earth can I have for lunch tomorrow?'
- Make your lunch with leftover dinner from the night before and put this into your planner (see page 141). For example, if on Monday you are having steak and salad, make yourself an extra serving of salad while you're making dinner and put it into a lunchbox then and there. Then you can add some cooked (or canned) chickpeas or butter beans for some starch and either cook a little extra steak for your lunchtime salad or pack a can of tuna or salmon to have with it.
- Make more of your dinner meal and take a portion to work the next day for your lunch. Frittatas are great for this; they make a great dinner served hot and a brilliant lunch served cold with salad – delicious.

You can of course use a mix-and-match approach with all these ideas if the thought of eating a variation on the same theme all week doesn't quite do it for you.

It comes down to planning and practice and, as ever, not giving up! You're on a journey.

YOU TIME: Do you struggle to eat well at work sometimes? If yes, tick here ☐

What is your new lunchtime plan?

_____

_____

_____

_____

_____

_____

_____

_____

_____

_____

_____

_____

_____

_____

_____

_____

OH NO, I FORGOT TO PACK MY LUNCH!

Don't you HATE that! You have gone to all that effort of making lunch and then you leave it in the fridge, or you just plain forget to pack yourself something. Fear not, everything is not lost and you really don't have an excuse to head out for a fat-packed lunch from your local bakery or café (as much as you may want to).

My suggestion is to have what I call a 'back-up' box, like the one in the car that I mentioned earlier. This is a box of food you keep at work that can be reached for in an emergency. The idea behind this is knowing that there aren't many healthy options available at the bakery or café, or perhaps you've had to stay late and just need something tasty to get you through to dinner.

If you spend a lot of time on the road and don't have a predictable timetable, it can be so useful to have a few things at hand in the car that are healthy options – far better than having to grab something unhealthy on the run (see page 175 for back-up boxes in the car).

Solution: back-up lunchbox

Here is what is in my emergency back-up lunchbox at work:

- Precooked rice (two-minute rice) – you can buy this in pouches or mini cups – and cans of tuna and salmon and, if you like them, sardines. These can be mixed together for a quick lunch.
- Cans or pots of heat-and-eat soup – go for ones with lots of veggies and some pulses if you can. Be mindful that these can be very high in salt, though.
- Wholegrain crackers – great with canned tuna or salmon on top.
- Mini-bags of nuts and seeds – these can be a good snack.
- Heat-and-eat pasta meals (ones that don't need to be refrigerated).

Do be mindful that these options are mostly low on the veggies compared with a standard healthy balanced lunch, so make sure you have extra veg at night to make up for it. They are also nowhere near as good for you as real whole foods, so best not to rely on this too often.

WARNING!

If you are a picker or like nibbling at food, having a stash too close at hand to your desk may tempt you into eating food just because it is there and, really, you don't need it. I have seen enough people put bags of dried apricots or nuts in their drawer at work for 'emergencies', then every day when they are feeling like a pick-me-up or are just a bit bored, they start munching away when they aren't hungry – and what they really needed was just five minutes of fresh air and daylight. If you are this person (and I was in previous years), keep food a little bit further away if you can.

YOU TIME: Do you need a back-up plan in case you forget your lunch? If yes, tick here ☐

What do you need to do to make sure this happens?

_____

_____

_____

_____

_____

_____

_____

_____

_____

WHAT TO DO WHEN EATING OUT IS PART OF YOUR WORK CULTURE

In some workplaces it is part of the normal culture to eat out at restaurants or cafés at lunchtime or to buy your lunch from a local shop or your onsite canteen and eat with your work buddies. Part of this is, in fact, very positive. It is a time when you get to talk about things other than work, build friendships and share stories with other people, and in my view that is important.

The flip-side, of course, depending on the situation, is that you can end up eating far more food (and kilojoules) than you need to and making decisions around food choices based on what other people want to do and not what is right for you.

Or it may be that you are required to go out for lunch as part of your job, such as building relationships with customers or other business. Remember, even if someone else is paying, it isn't free! If you are eating more than you need, you will have to burn those kilojoules off at some stage (and it may be hours at the gym) and it is also COSTLY in terms of your happiness.

When people go on a 'diet' or start following a special eating programme, it often means that they eat on their own, avoid eating with other people and see eating times as something to 'do' as part of a plan, rather than being able to enjoy eating. That is the last thing I want for you when you are trying to Lose Weight for Life! I don't want to see you hiding in a corner eating your special 'diet' food and becoming socially isolated – that isn't a long-term solution. However, neither do I want you to say 'Stuff it, I am just going to eat whatever I want to at work to be sociable' – that attitude will get you nowhere either and will keep unwanted kilos attached. So, time to find some middle ground.

Solution: eat well within your work culture

Here are my ideas to help you to enjoy eating at work and keep up your work relationships, without blowing out totally!

- Where possible, if you are going to have the odd lunch out or head to a café, see if you can make a suggestion about where to go, somewhere you know you can get healthy food which is an appropriate portion size. Don't just follow others – be proactive.
- Suggest a 'bring and share' lunch if you have a close group of work friends. Take it in turns to bring healthy lunches for your buddies and make the challenge for them to also bring in something healthy. If you have five people doing this, you would only need to make lunch one day a week.
- Take your lunch with you. If your colleagues all go out and buy their lunch, still go with them, so you aren't missing out on good conversations, but take your lunch with you and, provided they are eating outside of the shop they buy it from, just eat yours when they eat theirs. If they have an issue with this then they aren't really good friends, are they?

- If there is a staff canteen or somewhere at work that provides food, have a talk to the appropriate person to see if they are willing to start making healthy lunch options such as salads, healthy sandwiches and soup in the colder months. Well worth a try. Same goes for any snack foods at work – get rid of those 'honesty box' style biscuit and chocolate boxes and get fruit delivered. No one needs to be eating monster biscuits or chocolate bars at work every day.
- If you are eating out at a work lunch, having more courses, an extra wine or digging into dessert because everyone else is, it will only cost you in terms of your wellbeing. The way I see it, that FREE food is really expensive. So, only order and eat what you need. At lunch meetings, I often order a starter size of something and a side of veggies or salad – that is more than enough for that time of the day!
- Another thing to think about is what you drink. I have been to loads of lunches where the norm is to drink wine. Now, I LOVE wine, I really do, but drinking at lunchtime makes me tired and means I am totally unproductive for the rest of the afternoon. I only drink wine when I want to, not when other people want me to or try to pressure me. If someone thinks you are 'boring' or not taking part by not drinking, that says more about them and their issues than it does about you. If you are happy in yourself and able to confidently and firmly say (with a smile), 'No thanks, I am fine' and move swiftly on to another conversation, people will just leave you alone on this one.

You time: Does your work culture make it tricky to eat well sometimes? If yes, tick here ☐

What can you do to be proactive and make things healthier for you (and probably others, too)?

_____
_____
_____
_____
_____
_____
_____
_____
_____
_____
_____

HOW DO I STOP MUNCHING AT MORNING AND AFTERNOON TEA?

Is it just me, or have you noticed that muffins, cakes and biscuits seem to be getting bigger every time you see them? I was working from a café the other day and I saw a slice of cake that was literally the most ridiculously oversized wedge I have ever seen; and it would have been at least 4000 kJ (and it was $6 I might add – you used to be able to get a whole meal for that much).

I saw a lady order a slice and, much like most of us would do, even though she was probably feeling sick halfway through eating it, she pushed on and polished off the lot. We just don't like waste, do we? Generally speaking, we like to feel we are getting what we pay for, and at $6, I would have wanted to take the plate and fork too!

As you know, muffins and slices can be just massive – even the mini versions aren't really that mini and are probably more like what a normal serving used to be. Treat foods such as these, along with biscuits, snack bars, milky coffees, frappés and savouries, are now seen as the 'norm' for morning and afternoon teas. Many people I meet are having things like this at least a few times a week, if not every day, particularly if there is an onsite café at work or biscuits and muffins are served at morning work meetings.

Despite the normality of these foods in our current environment, please understand these are NOT at all everyday foods – and also be warned that muffins are really just cakes cooked in a muffin tin. Even if they are bran or 'low-fat' muffins, if they are the size of your hand they are likely to have more kilojoules than you need for a snack. So don't be fooled.

Solution: have a plan to manage morning and afternoon tea time

Sometimes we can end up eating food just because it is there or because it is what everyone else is doing, but when you are working on losing weight for life, you are working on being your own person when it comes to food, eating what your body needs and doing what is right for you.

Cake will always be around, as will muffins and biscuits. Don't fall into the trap of eating them every time you can. I only eat a cake or muffin very, very occasionally (every few months at most) and that is only when it is the best-looking slice of cake in the whole wide world and only if I will really truly enjoy every mouthful. I certainly don't dig into chocolate brownie made with compound chocolate or birthday cake every time there is a celebration, which in some workplaces can be as often as a few times a week. Not because I am trying to be holier than thou, but quite simply because now I actually know I don't enjoy those foods anymore – they aren't as good as people make them out to be, especially when you learn to have no emotional attachment to them.

Here's what you can do instead:

- Pack your own healthy snacks and encourage others to bring in healthy options for celebrations at work.

- Talk to those in charge of food choices at work and see if there is anything that can be done to make sure there is a balanced range of snack options available.
- If you feel you just can't control yourself around these foods, keep tuned – we will be looking at emotional attachment to foods later on (see page 198).

YOU TIME: Do you need to make better choices at morning and afternoon tea? If yes, tick here ☐

What do you need to do to make this happen?

_____

_____

_____

_____

_____

_____

_____

_____

_____

_____

_____

_____

_____

_____

_____

_____

_____

_____

HOW DO I MANAGE WHEN I AM SOCIALISING?

Some people believe that to lose weight you need to be boring, avoid everything you like and be what my brother describes as a 'fun sponge'. This couldn't be FURTHER from the truth. It is all about your attitude, your state of mind and being okay with having fun without over-indulging.

I am sure you have noticed that pretty much all social activities in some way, shape or form can revolve around food. Going out for dinner, dinner parties, going to the movies (eating popcorn and chocolate), watching the rugby (with beers, pies and chips), catching up for coffee and cake or a wine and some nibbles. Now, it is not that sharing food and drink is in any way a bad thing, it is great; but if you are a sociable person, it can be impossible to lose weight if everything you do revolves around food. So, let's look at some solutions.

Solution: eat well when socialising

- Organise healthy catch-ups with friends: go to a yoga class and then have a cuppa and chat at home; go for a walk – you can chat away, burning kilojoules at the same time; or go to regular gym classes with friends and catch up for a green tea afterwards.
- For social occasions which do revolve around food, make them healthy. Ditch the snacks to start with and just have a delicious main meal. Endless chips and dips every time you catch up with people aren't necessary. At a dinner party, make your entrée the nibbles people have when they arrive, rather than doubling up on starters.

YOU TIME: Do you need to make better choices when you are socialising? If yes, tick here ☐

What do you need to do to make this happen?

_____
_____
_____
_____
_____
_____
_____
_____
_____
_____

WHAT ABOUT WHEN THE NIBBLES COME OUT?

Damn chips and dips, they can taste so good, but are just so ridiculously un-helpful when you are watching your waistline. Once you start you can't stop, and it can be very difficult to know how much you have eaten. Often you end up eating more kilojoules than you would for a whole meal and you haven't even sat down at the table to eat your dinner yet.

Here are some insights for you (sorry, I know the truth is painful):

- 50 g of chippies (a big handful) = 1000 kJ, 15 g fat (that's a tablespoon of fat)
- 50 g of chippies and 3 tbsp of Kiwi dip = 1300 kJ, 21 g fat (that's 4 tablespoons of fat)
- 15 Snax crackers = 1050 kJ, 15 g fat
- 10 rice crackers with a slice of brie on top = 1400 kJ, 27 g fat

Solution: eat healthy nibbles

- If you are going to have nibbles, have a platter with vegetables (carrots, celery, cucumber, snow peas, blanched broccoli) and hummus, a low-fat yoghurt dip and a tomato salsa. Put out some olives, gherkins or some sundried tomatoes. Smoked salmon is also a little bit of luxury to add, if you like. If you are asked to bring food to someone else's place, look at taking something healthy then, too.
- If you are going to someone else's place where you know there will be chips and dips galore, don't arrive starving hungry. Once the first glass of wine has passed your lips, if you are peckish, the snacks will become irresistible. Have a salad, some soup or fruit and yoghurt before you go to fill the gap.
- Avoid sitting too close to temptation. It is a fact that the closer we sit to food, the more likely we are to eat it. If you arrive at someone's place and there are nibbles on the table, where possible position yourself so you are not within easy reach of the food – you will, I hope, eat less.

YOU TIME: Do you need to eat healthier nibbles? If yes, tick here ☐

What do you need to do to make this plan happen?

_____
_____
_____
_____
_____
_____
_____
_____
_____
_____

BUFFETS ARE A NIGHTMARE – HOW CAN I COPE?

Barbecues and buffet-style eating has got to be one of my favourite things. I love trying different foods and being able to serve myself. The only thing is that these 'pick what you like' feasts can be disastrous for overloading on food and eating more than you need to. Also, just remember that the more choices there are, the more you are likely to eat, and be mindful of the size of the plate you pick up – the bigger the plate, the bigger the portion.

Solution: make good buffet choices

- Choose a small- to medium-sized plate if you can, rather than the biggest one.
- Have a look at EVERYTHING that is laid out before you dig in. Start by filling your plate with the salad and vegetable stuff first (assuming, and fingers crossed, there is some). Try to fill half your plate with non-starchy veg or salad (minus those drowning in high-fat dressings). Then have a small serving of a few of your favourite (and healthier) options.
- No need to try everything; remember there will be other buffets and barbecues in your lifetime.
- Take your own healthier options to a barbecue if you are asked to take food. Salads, skinless chicken, lean meat, fish, prawns and other seafood are all delicious and good for you.

YOU TIME: Do you need to have a plan for dealing with buffets? If yes, tick here ☐

What do you need to do to make this plan happen?

_____

_____

_____

_____

_____

_____

_____

_____

_____

_____

EATING OUT – WHAT TO CHOOSE?

If you have a group of friends or a partner who just loves to eat out, I know it can be tricky to keep on track with your healthy eating plan – particularly if your friends/partner love creamy curries, pizza and like to top up your wine left, right and centre to ensure you are having a 'good time' . . . But fear not, here is what you can do.

Solution: eat well when eating out

- Where you can, try to involve yourself in choosing the restaurant (without being pushy and over-obsessive about it – there is NOTHING worse than someone who makes things difficult when you are going out to eat and picks at every little detail; people won't invite you again). I tend to suggest Japanese or places that I know serve salads and lighter main courses.
- Look at the menu online before you go and figure out what you might like to order.
- Order an entrée with a large side of veggies or a salad and have that as your 'main'. This is particularly useful in restaurants where portions are big.
- Ask for your dressing and sauces on the side where appropriate. If you need a recap of why, remember 2 tablespoons of mayonnaise, hollandaise, béarnaise or any high-fat creamy dressing has around the same number of kilojoules as a chocolate bar.
- Be the sober driver when you can; no alcohol is a great way to keep your kilojoules down – and you can still have fun.

YOU TIME: Do you need to make healthier choices when eating out? If yes, tick here ☐

What do you need to do to make this plan happen?

_____
_____
_____
_____
_____
_____
_____
_____
_____
_____
_____

MANAGING ALCOHOL

People often try to justify drinking because, in some way, they believe it is good for them, and I get that. If it was really true, I would probably do the same. Don't get me wrong; there are some good studies which suggest that for people of certain ages (older adults), a SMALL amount of alcohol (we are talking less than 2 units a day) can have a positive impact on heart health.

However, as alcohol is linked very strongly to cancers, mental illness, osteo-porosis, diseases of the liver and other chronic diseases, it is ludicrous to suggest that these potential small positive effects of drinking alcohol for some people is a justifiable reason to think that drinking is in some way 'good for you'. There are much better ways to promote optimal health and wellbeing which don't include alcohol. On top of that, alcohol is high in kilojoules and very unhelpful for those who want to be slim, fit and healthy.

Now, I enjoy drinking as much as the next person so I am not getting my big baton out here to make you feel bad by any means; but just be crystal clear that if you are drinking alcohol, you are doing so because you enjoy it and are totally aware of its impact on you (it is a toxin, after all), and not because you hope it is somehow going to make you live longer. If you don't drink alcohol, don't start because you think it will improve your health – stay as you are.

At the end of a busy and stressful day, it can be nice to head home, pour yourself a glass of wine or open a beer and relax. That is fine, provided it is an occasional thing rather than an everyday habit which has become part of your routine and your way of coping with the world. I have met so many people who, over time, get in the habit of opening a bottle of wine each night to help them chill out after a long day and either drink half or the whole bottle themselves – and that is only Monday to Friday, let alone what happens on the weekend.

NO judgement here because this has become a very 'normal' habit for many people, but it is one which needs addressing. Not only because a bottle of wine is near enough to 3400 kJ, but also because alcohol is a toxin and when it breaks down in the body it creates products which circulate in your system and stop you from getting a good night's sleep. Alcohol will indeed knock you out and possibly make you feel sleepy, but while you may sleep through the night after you have been drinking, the quality of this sleep will be poor. What that means is you will wake up not feeling rested, just tired and exhausted. This breeds a dangerous and vicious cycle of fatigue, stress and needing to open a bottle of wine when you get home to cope with the pressures of the day! See where I am going with this?

Facts on booze

- A standard-strength bottle of beer and a 150 ml glass of wine have roughly the same number of kilojoules.
- Cider is similar in kilojoules to beer – just with a tiny bit more sugar in some cases.
- Low-carb beer really is a bit of a waste of time; as I have already mentioned, regular beer isn't particularly high in carbs anyway, and the low-carb versions are only very slightly lower in kilojoules. My suggestion is to have less of the beer you like rather than digging into more low-carb beers thinking you are being healthier.
- Low-alcohol beers are lower in kilojoules than other beers so a better choice for the waistline.
- See pages 105–6 for guidelines on alcohol.

Solution: find ways to drink less

- Organise catch-ups with friends that don't always revolve around alcohol.
- Have at least two alcohol-free days a week – but ideally MANY more!
- If you are using alcohol to wind down every day or as a stress reliever, find an alternative – a hot bath, a pot of herbal tea, deep breathing or reading.
- If you are a white wine drinker or love beer or cider and want to cut down, avoid keeping chilled bottles in the fridge – it's much less appealing to tuck into a warm glass of sauvignon.
- If you drink spirits, measure out what you are having with a 30 ml shot glass – it can be surprising how much you have when you do a free pour.
- With spirits, use soda water as a mixer where you can. I have vodka, gin or rum with soda and lots of fresh lime or flavoured vodkas with soda. If you like, you can use a diet mixer which has no sugar or kilojoules.

YOU TIME: Do you need to address your drinking habits? If yes, tick here ☐

What do you need to do to make this happen?

MANAGING WHEN YOU'RE ON HOLIDAY

Once you have got things sorted, it can be pretty easy to stick to a weekly routine when it comes to your eating habits. But, heavens, what about holidays and weekend trips? It can be really easy to pack up your stuff and head on your way without giving a thought to what you are going to eat while you are away. Before you know it, you might be falling back into old habits: drinking more than you want to, grazing on chips and dips all afternoon, and skipping your daily serves of fruit and veg.

Now you don't for a minute need to plan to the ends of the earth when you go away, but wouldn't it be nice to still keep up most of your healthy habits and come back feeling even more fabulous and energised than before you left rather than returning with shorts that feel too tight and a bit of a muffin top?

Remember, losing weight for life is not about dieting, banning the foods that you like or not enjoying yourself. It is about helping you find ways to tip the balance so you can permanently eat well and have treats in small amounts and really enjoy them!

Solution: eat healthily on holiday

- Before you head away for the weekend or on a trip, go to the shops to pick up some healthy bits and pieces which you might not be able to get at your destination: fresh fruit, veggies, breakfast stuff and healthy snacks.
- If you have a long car journey ahead, stop somewhere nearer to your final destination to pick up some healthy bits and pieces – there might be a great fruit store on the way (there are so many in New Zealand), or stop at the supermarket which is near to where you are staying.
- If you are heading somewhere on a plane, see if you can find out where a local food store is close to where you are staying, so you can pick up some basics.
- If you are planning to drink spirits, get some soda water or diet mixers to take with you (if you are driving, of course, and have room in the car). In my experience, when you get to the more remote places around the country you can often only find full-sugar drinks and hardly ever soda water.
- If you are staying in self-catering accommodation while you are away, stock up on salad stuff and fruit, and take a few healthy recipes with you.
- When you come back after a trip away or a weekend break, Sunday night dinner can often end up as a takeaway because you don't have anything in. Instead, get some fresh filled pasta from the supermarket and have it in the fridge all ready for when you come home to have with frozen veggies. Alternatively, eggs can make a great meal: eggs and beans on toast or an omelette are quick throw-together dinners. See page 142 for suggestions on other back-up meals for when you get back from holiday.

YOU TIME: Do you need to make plans for healthier holidays? If yes, tick here ☐

What do you need to do to make this plan happen?

_____
_____
_____
_____
_____
_____

BORED OF EATING THE SAME OLD THING?

There is nothing worse than eating the same old boring meals. It is totally ironic, really, when there are hundreds of TV shows, endless food magazines and recipe books and more than 300 million recipes on the internet, that most of us end up cooking the same five to ten recipes each and every week.

We are creatures of habit. Trying new things takes time and effort and is also a risk. What if the recipe doesn't turn out right? What if you don't have the particular herb or spice needed? What if the kids won't eat it?

The fact is that regardless of how many recipes there are, we all often eat a limited number of things. This really proves my point that just because the knowledge is there, it doesn't necessarily change what we do! We need systems and processes to integrate what we know into new everyday habits.

Solution: make your meals interesting

- Get onto meal planning – see page 141.
- Try one new recipe each week and make it a set night of the week so you know to include this in your plan and you can communicate this to anyone else who is cooking or who you are cooking for. Make it a night of the week when you are likely to have a bit more time, maybe mid-week or even on a Saturday or Sunday.
- Make yourself a recipe bible. This is NOT a book shoved full of all the lovely recipes you would 'one day' like to make, because we all have those and, much like recipe books, you never make anything from them! When you have tried a new dish, and it works and you know you will have the ingredients in for this recipe, and you also know that it will be something quick and easy to make on regular occasions and that everyone likes it, then and ONLY then can it be added to your recipe bible (just a folder with those plastic sleeves is fine). You can then use this to help you plan your weekly menu and shopping list, knowing that the ideas you have in the book work well and are easy to make.

YOU TIME: Do you want to make your meals more interesting? If so, tick here ☐

What do you need to do to make this plan happen?

_____
_____
_____
_____
_____
_____
_____
_____
_____
_____
_____
_____
_____

I'M SICK OR INJURED AND CAN'T POSSIBLY EXERCISE – HELLO CHOCOLATE!

Most people will get some kind of cough, cold or feel under the weather at some point during the year – be it the flu or perhaps you have pulled a muscle and can't exercise as you normally would. This is the perfect time for some of your 'excuses' to crop up again and for you to justify eating rubbish. But you and I both know this is only temporarily relieving the pain. Doing this sets you back in the long run and is likely to only make you feel worse about yourself on top of your cold/flu/injury – it's not a winning combo. Make a decision to be kind to yourself and to help yourself.

Solution: manage sickness and injury

- If you are sick, have a cold or the flu, see if you can get someone to pick you up some healthy snacks including fresh fruit, veggies and soups.
- If your appetite isn't the best, have small snack-size meals which are still packed with nutrients: a small bowl of cereal with milk, chopped banana with some walnuts and yoghurt, home-made popcorn (without sugar, salt or butter), edamame beans or scrambled egg on a slice of toast.
- If you fancy something sweet, go for some yoghurt blended with frozen berries and a teaspoon of honey or make yourself some custard with low-fat milk, less sugar than normal and serve a sliced banana on top.

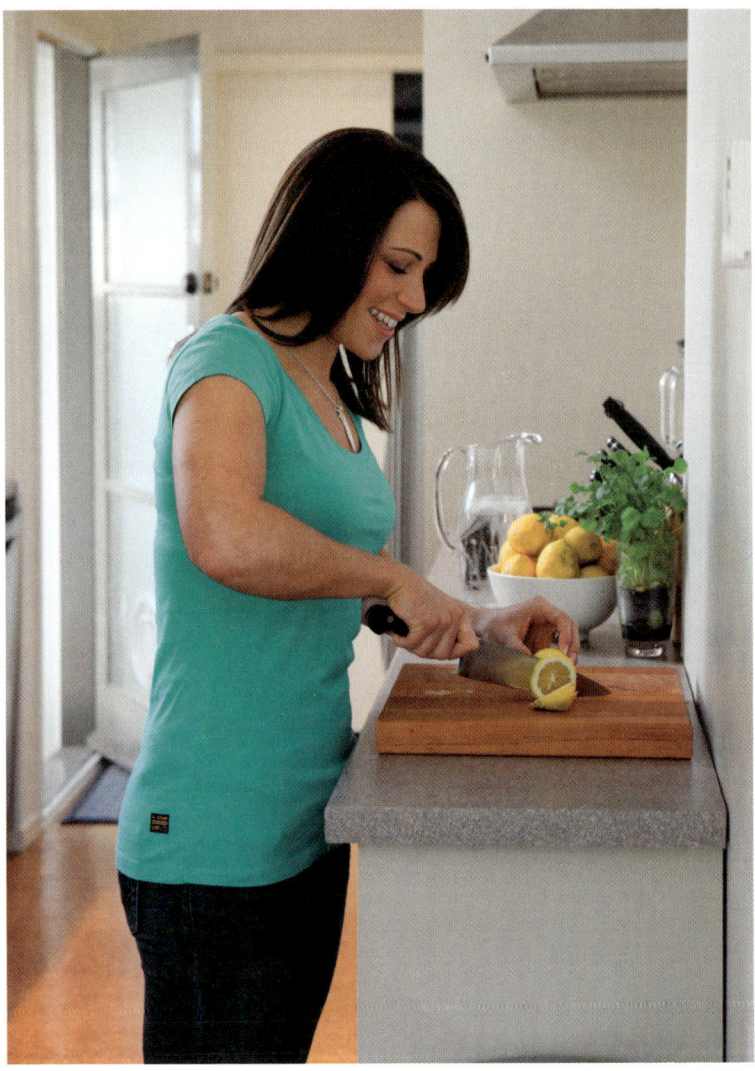

- Keep up your fluids when you aren't feeling well – it can be all too easy to forget about this. Herbal teas are fantastic if you are looking for something hot. Chai tea is great with a teaspoon of honey if you are wanting something a little sweet. Or try hot water with lemon juice and honey.
- If you are injured, check with your GP or physio to see if there is anything you are able to do to keep active, even if it isn't the usual thing you do. Maybe you can still walk, swim, aqua-jog or do work on your upper or lower body at the gym without creating any issues for your injured area.

IS SOMEONE SABOTAGING YOUR SUCCESS?

I hate to break this to you, but you may also find that someone is sabotaging your weight-loss journey. It won't necessarily be a deliberate thing, but I am really sorry to tell you that it is incredibly common to find that someone you know, probably someone you know very well, may be making it difficult for you to stick to your goals. Do any of these comments ring a bell with you?

- 'Go on, one slice of cake won't hurt you!'
- 'Let's go out and grab a coffee and maybe a muffin, too; we deserve to treat ourselves.'
- 'I have baked your favourite biscuits; you have to have one.'
- 'I will bring some chocolate home; I think we need it after today!'

Has anyone said something like this to you before? Something that makes you feel like you are being led away from your goal rather than heading towards it?

It is a terrible truth (particularly with women) that sometimes we sabotage other people's success or weight-loss goals. If you are honest with yourself, you may have done it to someone else before.

So, why does this happen? It is not because you or your friend or partner is a horrible person, it is just very hard for them to see you losing weight successfully when they aren't at a point when they can do it themselves, or simply that they feel threatened by you changing.

So, subconsciously, without any malicious intent, they will try to sabotage your success, expose your weaknesses and encourage you to go off track to make themselves feel better about the fact that they aren't ready to change or for you to change.

There are also the cases when someone might say to you, 'I really feel like a glass of wine, but I can't have one if you aren't drinking.' Sound familiar? A lot of people feel uncomfortable eating or drinking something considered naughty or a treat food on their own; it makes them feel guilty. If you go along with it, you are relieving them of the guilt.

Solution: work on your relationship with food

Before you file for divorce or dump your best friend, remember a lot of this is subconscious and they aren't doing it to hurt you. They just haven't dealt with their issues – but, as harsh as it sounds, that is their problem, not yours.

What you can do is work on your own relationship with food and look at creating habits and behaviours which help you reach your goals. Your job in this world is not to relieve other people's guilt by damaging yourself and my advice is not to eat food or have a drink because other people want you to. If you really think about it, you aren't helping yourself, or them.

Ideally, there shouldn't be guilt around food, even wine, chocolate and other treats. You should be able to include these in small amounts and really enjoy them. To do this, you need to disregard the notion that food is somehow 'good or bad' – after all, it's just food. But some of us need to unpack our emotional responses to food. And that brings us to the next section.

Part 4: When food has messed with your mind

Food messing with your mind

DEALING with food used for the wrong purpose:

Emotional eating

Self-sabotage

Eating for comfort

Eating for punishment

For some people, food is just food. It is the fuel and nourishment that the body needs to make it function and that, quite simply, is that. For those who see food in this light (including my husband), it is common for them to enjoy eating and drinking without guilt, to stop eating when they are full and they find it impossible to even conceptualise that you could in some way have an emotional relationship with bread, ice cream or cake – after all, it is just food, isn't it?

Do you know someone like this? How lucky they are, living in a blissful existence where food is just, well, food. For the rest of us, to varying degrees, food can have so much more meaning. Food can control the way you think, the way you feel and can have the ability to make or break your day – how irritating!

So, why is that? Because of specific experiences and circumstances, eating and drinking can become linked with certain emotions and, over time, food is given meaning and power – and sometimes it seems that it can control you.

Here are some examples of what I mean:

- It could be that you were given dessert or ice cream when you were good and it was taken away if you were naughty – you learnt that food was linked to how you behaved.
- If you have been on and off diets your whole life, you may see certain foods as 'good' or 'bad' and feel guilty when you eat too many bad foods.
- You may have got yourself into a cycle of semi-starving and then bingeing when you have a bad day or something goes wrong and you just don't know how to eat normally anymore.

All these things (and so many hundreds and thousands more) can have an impact on the way you feel about food and the role food plays in your life. Whatever you have been through, and whatever issues you now face, the truth is that if food is not just fuel and nourishment to be enjoyed, you are likely to be using food for something food wasn't designed for! If this is the case, food may seem to have some kind of power over you, and even though you should technically be able to control what you put in your mouth, it doesn't feel like that at all. Fear not, though, this is my area of passion and interest in a big way, and I have some solutions coming up. First, though, let's work out how food may have messed with your mind.

A DYSFUNCTIONAL RELATIONSHIP WITH FOOD

Last night I was at a dinner function and got chatting about food to a lovely lady sitting next to me. We got onto the topic of eating behaviour and she confessed to me that even though she was a very healthy weight and size she had a very dysfunctional relationship with food and had never really known who to talk to about it. She had gone on diets when she was younger, but realised they weren't really long-term solutions. In the last five or so years (she was in her fifties) she had taken a new approach: trying to be really 'good' and strict six days a week and having one day when she ate whatever she liked and had a blow-out if she wanted. She didn't see this as a diet as such, just a way to cope and keep her weight in check – fair play, I guess. However, there was still a problem. Even though her approach did kind of work in terms of keeping her food intake in check, she had really got this notion of food being 'good' and 'bad' stuck in her head. She described to me the awful days when she felt like she had eaten a bit too much the day before, so tried to hardly eat anything that day so she wouldn't gain weight but then, without really knowing why, she ended up bingeing at random times of the day. It wasn't always on junk food, but there were times when she just couldn't stop eating once she had started.

There are so many examples of dysfunctional relationships with food and you don't have to be underweight or overweight to struggle with these issues. I meet people every single day who you would think from looking at them that they have nothing to worry about when it comes to food. They are a healthy weight and size and look okay, and yet these same people worry every minute of every day about food and situations involving food. They just can't seem to escape their own minds – and it is making them miserable. I was one of those people. I know this life all too well – it's not pretty.

Whether you can't commit to full meals and pick all day, starve and then binge, spit your food out after eating (more common than you might think), eat in private when you are meant to be on a 'diet' or have major anxiety when it comes to eating out or sharing food with other people – do not panic! I have met SO many people who give themselves a really hard time about these things, because they feel like their behaviour is stupid, illogical and that they should be able to stop it. Let me reassure you, you are NOT stupid, dumb, ridiculous or different. All that has happened is that somewhere along the way food has acquired power, meaning and control over you. There are solutions though. You don't need to live like this forever, I promise.

Eating for comfort

It is very common to use food or drink to comfort yourself after a hard day, when something has gone wrong or you just need cheering up. Food tastes delicious, it doesn't judge you for whatever just happened and, while you are eating it, it can make you feel amazing. Problem is, you are using food for something that it wasn't designed for. You are likely to be eating when you are not hungry and using food to help control the way you feel. The aftermath in many cases also isn't great; you may have feelings of guilt, disappointment and self-hatred for what you have just done, particularly if you are trying to lose weight and by comfort-eating you are taking yourself away from your vision, your goal, your dream.

Once again, though, you aren't mad, stupid or odd for doing this; you have just learnt to use food (or drink) as the default coping mechanism in times of stress. What you need to do is find a new coping mechanism that isn't as damaging, as well as working on your thinking at the times when you feel like using food to comfort yourself.

Eating for punishment

At a meeting last week I was talking about how people use food for punishment and everyone in the room looked at me blankly (to be fair, they were all foodies who had no attachment to food other than for fuel and its tastiness). This experience raised an interesting point for me. People commonly only talk about eating for comfort, but from my own experiences, and those of many clients I have worked with, food can equally be used as punishment and a tool of self-harm.

If food can control the way you feel, as well as your weight and size, when you are mad at yourself, don't feel good enough or disappointed, you may actually eat large volumes of food that you don't really need or want, not for comfort but rather as a form of punishment.

In my experience, those of us who use food as a form of self-harm don't always seem to reach for the chocolate and sweet treats, but often binge on foods such as dry crackers or cereal, have triple helpings at meals and sometimes eat large amounts of food they don't even really like. It is a really useful exercise to look at the times when you eat more than you need to and see if there is any difference between times when you may eat for punishment rather than comfort. To some people this will make no sense at all, but I bet you there will be many of you reading this right now, thinking, 'Wow, she is a mind reader.' I know because I have been there, just like you.

HOW TO MANAGE WHEN FOOD HAS MESSED WITH YOUR MIND

First up, to overcome a dysfunctional relationship with food, you need to accept that what you are doing right now and some of the funny things you do around food aren't 'wrong' or 'bad', and you are not a terrible failure for having these issues. You are NORMAL! Once you have stopped giving yourself a hard time, you can move on to finding a solution to what I like to call bumps in the road or triggers – these are things which get in the way of your Lose Weight for Life journey. These bumps just need to be found, explored and worked on – from there, the future is bright and beautiful.

So, it is time for you to get out the pen and paper again – let's get clear on what has been going on!

1. Identify the issue

What we are looking for here are all the times, situations and circumstances (the bumps or triggers) when you are eating more than you know you need to or want to be eating. These may be times when you are eating for comfort, punishment, reward, bingeing, picking, nibbling or whatever feels like an issue for you.

At the moment, what is likely to be happening is that whenever one of these bumps or triggers comes up, without realising it (and without really thinking you have a choice), you end up eating or drinking something you either don't really want, don't need or are having for all the wrong reasons. It's a bit like this:

Bump/trigger

→ Situations
→ Circumstances   Default behaviour →   **Outcome**
→ Thoughts/feelings   Eating/drinking

You may have identified some of these bumps or triggers in the previous section of the book – that is fine. Here we are looking to delve a little deeper into why you struggle with these times in particular.

Here are some examples of bumps and triggers:

- When I argue with my boyfriend/girlfriend/husband/wife I get so upset that afterwards I hit the chocolate or something sweet.
- As soon as my kids leave for school, I feel like I am on my own and lonely. I start picking at food in the cupboard to take the lonely feeling away.
- I hate my job and when my boss is rude to me during the day, I end up heading home via the drive-through and picking up whatever I feel like – but always more than I know I need.
- When I have one biscuit, I feel really guilty and because I am trying to lose weight I feel like a failure. For some reason, though, I then eat the whole packet rather than stopping at just one.
- I don't eat proper meals but pick at bits here and there, and have little slices of cake at a time. I probably end up eating more than a normal slice of cake by the time I have nibbled my way through the smaller pieces. I am too scared to eat big meals.

- I find it hard to eat with other people. I have super-strict control of my portions and what I eat every day, but when I am on my own at the weekend, I pick all day long and often end up in a bingeing cycle. Sometimes I vomit afterwards.
- When I feel I have done well or achieved something good, I will end up hitting the wine and chocolate as a reward for my efforts.

There are endless times when you may eat more than you need or want to, but really focus on the main ones, the times when you have the biggest problems, the ones that really bother and irritate you. If you aren't quite sure of your 'problem' times, you may want to keep a diary of what you eat and how you feel for a week or so to see if you can identify the specific triggers.

For most people I have worked with, they tend to have five or six key bumps or triggers. You really need to work out what these situations are because if you aren't 100 per cent aware of them, you can't do anything to change them. Clarity is essential.

YOU TIME: Identify the issue

On a piece of paper, draw yourself a blank table with six columns and seven rows (which includes one for your headings). Label each column as outlined below and then start by filling in column **A. Situation** with your key problem times when food messes with your mind.

A. Situation	B. Rename	C. The details	D. New thoughts	E. New default behaviour	F. Making your environment supportive of change

Remember: NO judgement on this please – that will only fuel the cycle of self-sabotage.

2. Rename your bump and trigger times

Once you have your KEY bump and trigger times I would like you to rename them, so whenever these times come up from now on, you instantly recognise them. When you are able to see the situation in black and white, you have the power to think and do something differently.

So, using my examples below, think about renaming your own situations:

A. Situation	B. Rename
When I argue with my boyfriend/girlfriend/ husband/wife I get so upset that afterwards I hit the chocolate or something sweet.	Argument mode
As soon as my kids leave for school, I feel like I am on my own and lonely. I start picking at food in the cupboard to take the lonely feeling away.	Feeling lonely
I hate my job and when my boss is rude to me during the day, I end up heading home via the drive-through and picking up whatever I feel like – but always more than I know I need.	Work irritation
When I have one biscuit, I feel really guilty and because I am trying to lose weight I feel like a failure. For some reason, though, I then eat the whole packet rather than stopping at just one.	Biscuit time
I don't eat proper meals but pick at bits here and there, and have little slices of cake at a time. I probably end up eating more than a normal slice of cake by the time I have nibbled my way through the smaller pieces. I am too scared to eat big meals.	Pick, pick, pick
I find it hard to eat with other people. I have super-strict control of my portions and what I eat every day, but when I am on my own at the weekend, I pick all day long and often end up in a bingeing cycle. Sometimes I vomit afterwards.	Binge time
When I feel I have done well or achieved something good, I will end up hitting the wine and chocolate as a reward for my efforts.	Didn't I do well!

YOU TIME: Rename your bump and trigger times

It doesn't matter how silly the names you come up with are – they are just something that you will be able to identify with very quickly when you are in the situation. Once you have thought of a new name for each bump/trigger time, go back to your blank table and fill in column **B. Rename**.

3. Digging into the detail

It is now time to go into a little more detail. Look at each of your bumps and triggers and answer the following questions about each of them:

- What are you thinking? You MUST answer this question. Take as long as you need to write something down about the thoughts that are going through your head when you're in this situation.
- How do you feel at the time this is happening?
- What are you hoping to get out of eating at this time? Relief? Pleasure? Punishment?
- What kinds of foods are you eating? Where do you get them from?

Based on my examples, think about how you would answer these questions:

A. Situation	C. The details
When I argue with my boyfriend/girlfriend/ husband/wife I get so upset that afterwards I hit the chocolate or something sweet.	• Thinking I am all alone and hopeless. • Feeling rejected, unloved and useless. • I want the pain to go away and sweet foods seem like the perfect solution. I tend to buy chocolate from the local shop or have ice cream from the freezer at home.
As soon as my kids leave for school, I feel like I am on my own and lonely. I start picking at food in the cupboard to take the lonely feeling away.	• Thinking that no one really loves me. • Feeling lonely and abandoned. • Wanting food to provide comfort and support. • Eating anything – salty and sweet – that is open in the fridge or pantry; I don't open new packets though.
I hate my job and when my boss is rude to me during the day, I end up heading home via the drive-through and picking up whatever I feel like – but always more than I know I need.	• Thinking I hate my job and being treated so badly, I might as well eat to make myself feel better. • Thinking that I'm scared of confronting my boss and working out a solution – I might get fired and I won't be able to find another job. • Feeling like I have no control over my life and I hate that other people make me feel like this. • Food is like a punishment for me being so useless and helpless. • Wanting salty fast food – I know it is bad for me. It's always from a drive-through.

A. Situation	C. The details
When I have one biscuit, I feel really guilty and because I am trying to lose weight I feel like a failure. For some reason, though, I then eat the whole packet rather than stopping at just one.	• Thinking that I have no will-power, I know what I need to do but can't do it, I am useless. • Also thinking, well, I have failed now by eating one biscuit, I might as well keep going, I deserve to feel like this. • Feeling bored, lonely and rejected. • Always have biscuits in the house because of the kids so I can't escape them.
I don't eat proper meals but pick at bits here and there, and have little slices of cake at a time. I probably end up eating more than a normal slice of cake by the time I have nibbled my way through the smaller pieces. I am too scared to eat big meals.	• Thinking that I will get fat if I eat too much, so best not to have big meals. • I need to be thinner to be happy. • Feeling out of control and can't stop thinking about food. • I end up getting hungry and then endlessly picking at food. I probably have more kilojoules in the end by doing this but can't see another way out. • I pick at bread, crackers, cake, baking – anything starchy really.
I find it hard to eat with other people. I have super strict control of my portions and what I eat every day, but when I am on my own at the weekend, I pick all day long and often end up in a bingeing cycle. Sometimes I vomit afterwards.	• Thinking that I can't control myself and can't trust myself. • I am not good enough. • Feeling scared of food – it has so much control over my mind and I hate it, I just can't stop thinking about it. • I don't ever eat from a plate. It tends to be worse when I am home on my own. • No specific foods, just whatever is around; even if I don't really like it, I eat it.
When I feel I have done well or achieved something good, I will end up hitting the wine and chocolate as a reward for my efforts.	• Thinking I deserve it and need a treat. • Feeling excited and like I need to celebrate. • Will celebrate on my own mostly, if I am honest – I eat and drink in private in most cases.

YOU TIME: Digging into the detail

Time to get down to the nitty gritty. Think about the questions at the start of this step. Now go to your blank table and fill in column **C. The details** with your own answers.

4. How can you change your thoughts?

Now that you are very clear on what you are thinking and doing at each of these bump or trigger times, you have put the power back in your hands. You can change your default eating and drinking habits and as a result get the outcome you want.

This is how you do it:

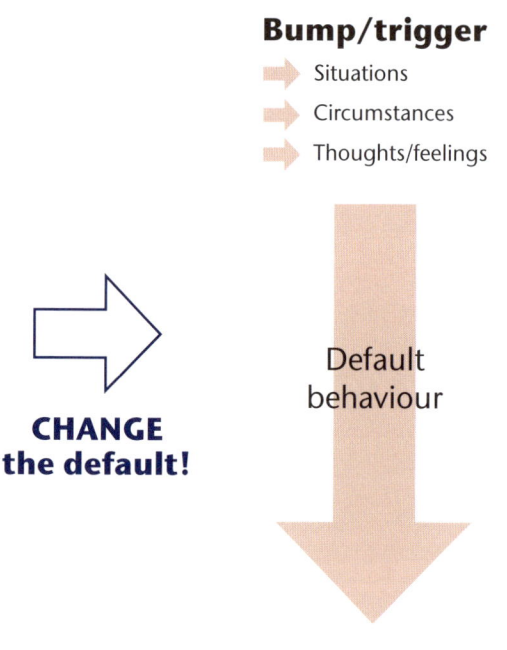

Bump/trigger

Situations

Circumstances

Thoughts/feelings

Default behaviour

CHANGE the default!

New positive OUTCOME

So, for each situation, bump or trigger time, come up with a new thought – a better thought that will help you when you are in the situation

Let's look at this example from a woman called Jane.

> I hate my job and when my boss is rude to me during the day, I end up heading home via the drive-through and picking up whatever I feel like – but always more than I know I need.

Jane's original thought was: 'I hate my job and being treated so badly, so I might as well eat to make myself feel better.'

Jane's new thought could be: 'I am upset and food will help me feel better, but only temporarily – I deserve to treat myself better.'

Here are some top tips for choosing your 'new' thoughts from a very good friend of mine, Louise Thompson, who is both a wellness coach and all-round fabulous woman.

Hello lovely readers!

I am so thrilled to be able to share some of the coaching tools I use with my clients with you to enhance the amazing journey Claire is taking you on in this book.

This is what I want you to know: your thoughts are super powerful. Your thoughts determine how you feel and how you behave. Your thoughts literally make your world. If you are overeating or carrying extra weight it's because you have thoughts that will lead you to that outcome. If you have healthier, more balanced thoughts you will have a healthier, more balanced body. It's pretty much that simple.

Simple but not easy! It takes time and practice to break down your thought patterns and beliefs, but it is SO worth it.

We are taught in school WHAT to think, but we are never taught HOW to think. And there is a big difference. When we just accept that all the thoughts that whiz through our minds are the truth, then we are at the mercy of our thoughts, which can then lead us to a whole heap of behaviours we don't really want, like overeating.

The very cool thing to know is that YOU HAVE THE POWER TO CHOOSE WHAT THOUGHTS YOU THINK.

Just like you have the power to choose what food you put into your body, you (yes, you) have the choice as to what thoughts you put into your mind. If you feed your mind with healthy thoughts you will get the body and the weight you want.

There is a whole book here in itself, but in a nutshell one of the things I coach clients to do is to be able to choose better-feeling thoughts and change their relationship with their body, self-esteem and food. In Claire's example opposite, the key thought in that scenario is not that Jane and her boss disagreed, it's the fact she thought 'I am being treated badly' about that interaction. This will lead to a thought like 'It's not fair' or 'I can't change it' or 'I hate my job'. These are all painful thoughts and they don't feel good. We don't like feeling painful thoughts. So, what many of us do is AVOID that painful thought by overeating or drinking. When we overeat or drink our mind becomes filled with thoughts such as 'I shouldn't have eaten that, I'm such a pig' and . . . da-dah . . . the problem of the painful thought is immediately solved because it is blocked by an avalanche of thoughts about what we have just eaten, our lack of willpower or self-control. We forget about hating the job because we are so busy hating ourselves! Relief, yes, but at a cost to our bodies, waistline and self-esteem.

However, if you take control of your thinking in this situation you can make a different choice. Know that WE CAN ONLY HOLD ONE THOUGHT IN OUR MINDS AT A TIME. So make it a good one. Instead of blocking the painful thought with another thought that also makes us feel bad ('I can't believe I just pigged out like that'), REPLACE THE ORIGINAL THOUGHT WITH A BETTER-FEELING THOUGHT.

So, again, based on the example above, by changing what Jane thinks, the outcome is changed.

So right now what is happening is this:

Jane has a disagreement with her boss and thinks 'I'm being treated badly'. She blocks that thought by overeating and thinking about how much she hates herself for overeating.

But she could change this by looking at her original thought.

Jane has a disagreement with her boss and thinks 'I'm being treated badly' but then realises that thought leads to overeating and so she chooses to pick a better-feeling thought such as 'Hmm . . . my boss was cross about that thing, but it's not a reflection on me. He was just having a bad day. It happens.' She then feels calm/detached/gratitude (any other positive emotion instead of upset) and therefore neutralises the need for her to avoid the pain by using food – a much better outcome.

You have probably realised that I am using the word **CHOOSE** a lot here. That repetition is deliberate. It's about a choice to own what you think and own what you feel. You can choose to feel that painful feeling (and there is no feeling so painful it can't be survived) and therefore the need to escape it with food, or you can choose to reach for a better-feeling thought that will still apply to that situation but means you don't need to overeat.

Every time we overeat it's an amazing opportunity to get to know ourselves better and to be kinder to ourselves. When we overeat, examining what has triggered that urge and what the painful thoughts are that we are trying to escape from through food is the key to finding our freedom with our relationship with food and weight. Find the thought and identify the feeling. Choose to simply replace the thought with a better one! You can only hold one thought in your mind at a time, so feed your mind with top-quality thoughts that bring you peace and calm, or at the least, less distress. The need to escape your thoughts and emotions through food will dissipate.

When you change the thought to a better-feeling thought you will find that changing your default behaviour is far easier. You will be bringing far more awareness to your true mental and emotional state, and switching to a more supportive default behaviour that is aligned to your goals is way easier.

Changing up your thoughts takes some practice and commitment but it will make an enormous impact on your relationship with food, with yourself and your overall wellbeing. It also means that the days of yo-yo dieting are gone forever.

Good luck! You can do it.

Louise

Louise Thompson is a life coach and yoga instructor (www.positivebalance.co.nz)

YOU TIME: Changing your thoughts

Look at your bump and trigger time thoughts. What new thoughts could you have? Once you have come up with a new, positive thought, fill in column **D. New thoughts** in your own table.

5. Doing something different

So, now that you have a better understanding of why you need to change what you think, let's also consider the need to change what you DO.

Using the example of the drive-through situation again, what could this person DO differently when this trigger time arises?

New options for coping when this situation arises:

- Texting or calling a friend straight away for a chat when you feel angry about work. You will need to be very specific about which friend, have their number at the top of your phone list and communicate with them so they know you need their support.
- Change the route you drive home so you are unable to go past a drive-through and plan your meals for the week so you know you have something tasty to look forward to when you get home.
- Leave money or credit cards in the boot of your car so you can't easily pay for the drive-through.

What you choose to do differently needs to be something quick, easy and totally feasible in that situation. For example, there is no point saying you will go for a walk when someone is mean to you at work if you don't really have time to leave the office! Texting someone, emailing someone, looking at a photo or reading something positive would be more appropriate.

What you choose to DO differently will completely depend on the nature of your bump or trigger. Here is a list of ideas which you could apply to your situation. I hope you will be able to come up with some of your own solutions. You need to make sure that what you choose to do is realistic and right for you and the situation.

- Head out for a walk – have your trainers and walking gear out and ready to go.
- Make a cup of green/herbal tea.
- Run a bath.
- Have a shower.
- Text a specific friend or family member.
- Take 10 deep breaths.
- Write down how you are feeling – get it all out on paper.
- Create a vision board with photos, words and images of where

you are going with your life, and when the difficult time arises go to that vision board and be assured that this situation is only temporary.

- Pick up a magazine and read something funny or light-hearted.
- Eat something small but filling before you go out to a buffet so you aren't starving and feel the need to eat everything.
- Commit to only eating off a plate or out of a bowl at all times.
- Be the sober driver every second weekend.
- Have low-kilojoule non-alcoholic drinks in the house to have when you get home from work or get into the habit of putting the kettle on and having a brew instead of a glass of wine.

Again, based on my examples, here is what I have come up with:

B. Rename	D. New thoughts	E. New default behaviour
Argument mode	'I choose to discuss what is bothering me rather than burying it in food. I'm not hungry, I am actually angry.'	Take 10 deep breaths and have a cup of tea.
Feeling lonely	'I am not hungry right now but I am feeling a little lonely. I am choosing to call my friend Sarah as that will lift my mood.'	Call your friend Sarah; if she is not around, write to her – even if you just scribble it down. You don't need to send it, just let the feelings come out.
Work irritation	'There were three things I enjoyed about my day and I am going to focus on those' or 'I'm going to meet with my boss tomorrow and see if we can figure out a solution to this. Eating a family bag of chips will not make my job better but I can have conversations that will.'	Drive a different way home, not via the drive- through.
Biscuit time	'I'm not actually hungry right now, I'm just wanting to unwind. I'm going to choose to go for a walk/play tennis/read a magazine instead.'	Pick up your magazine and read at least a few pages with a cup of herbal tea.

B. Rename	D. New thoughts	E. New default behaviour
Pick, pick, pick	'I love and trust my body. It's okay to enjoy eating when I am hungry as long as I stop when I am satisfied.'	Eat only from a plate or bowl at the table with cutlery every time. Commit to eating everything mindfully.
Binge time	'I am normal and I can trust myself. I have the power to choose foods which nourish my body and I can stop when I am full.'	Make a plan for the weekend so you know what you will be eating, and as part of that have one small treat which you share with a friend, and really enjoy it without guilt.
Didn't I do well!	'Yay me! I am going to choose to celebrate by buying those awesome shoes/booking a spa day/whatever feels like a treat but doesn't involve food.'	Start a bank account or have a money jar which you add cash to when you have done well and want to celebrate.

YOU TIME: Doing something different

Have a good think about what you DO when a bump or trigger time arises. Once you are very clear on what it is that you do, think – what could you do that is different? What can you change to make sure you aren't sabotaging yourself? Write down your ideas in column **E. New default behaviour.**

6. Making your environment supportive of change

To make sure you are able to follow through with your new default thoughts and behaviours, you will need to come up with a plan to ensure your environment supports your new plans. There is no point planning to make yourself a cup of tea rather than pouring a glass of wine when you get home from a stressful day, if there are always going to be open bottles of wine in the fridge, chilled and ready to drink, and a wine glass on the bench which acts as a visual reminder of your old habits.

Take time to think about the things which might make it tricky to stick to your new plan. What might get in the way? What do you need to change about your environment to make sure you can do what, deep down, you really want to do (eat and drink for the right reasons)? So, with my examples:

Argument mode

You are planning to take deep breaths and have a cup of tea rather than dig into something sweet. To be able to do this, you need to make sure there aren't huge amounts of sweet foods kept in the house and that you don't end up going home via the dairy to buy chocolate. How can you make sure this doesn't happen? Maybe committing to buying less sweet foods; no one needs them in the house. Don't have cash readily available when you pass the dairy.

Feeling lonely

Here, rather than picking at food in the pantry you are going to call your friend. To make sure this happens, you may also need to rearrange your pantry so snack foods are out of sight or stop buying them in the first place. You could also put healthy chopped-up veggies at the front of your fridge in case, at the beginning, you do go into some kind of default picking mode. These are better than sugary, salty, fatty snacks. Third, you will need to let Sarah know you may be calling her in times of need and put her number at the top of your phone list.

Work irritation

You are planning to go home by a different route, not via the drive-through. You will also need to make sure that you plan your meals and have something tasty to look forward to for dinner when you get home or, no doubt, you will pick up fast food anyway.

Biscuit time

If you plan to read a magazine and have a cuppa rather than eat biscuits, you will need to make sure you have a magazine that you want to read (you could start a subscription). It is also a good idea to find a teapot and some tea you really like to make the whole experience of sitting down and drinking more enjoyable. Also, best to get rid of the biscuits if they are that much of an issue for you – the kids can learn to live without them.

Pick, pick, pick

If it has been years since you sat down and had a proper meal, it might seem strange at first to do this. To help ease the transition, get yourself a plate and bowl or crockery you really like. Buy yourself a placemat and, when you can, sit down and eat at the table with nice surroundings. If you are at work, try to do the same; be sure you alter your environment so you are able to sit down and commit to eating.

Binge time

If you know things always go pear-shaped at the weekend, make yourself a little plan. Work out where you will be and what you might be eating. Head to the market and get some fresh fruit and veggies to make some new and interesting healthy meals which you can freeze for the week ahead. Plan a walk, bike ride or something active with a friend every weekend, too. Get yourself into a better routine.

Didn't I do well!

If your plan is to save up and buy yourself something nice, you will still need to cope with the fact that part of you will be looking for instant gratification. If you eat and drink in private, try to avoid having fatty, sugary foods around which will be all too easy to eat. Celebrate by cooking yourself a nice dinner and inviting a friend over, too, so you can share the celebration.

Other things you might want to think about to ensure your environment supports change:

- Do you need a picture on your wall, phone or in your wallet to remind you of your new plan?
- Do you need to talk to someone and let them know you might call/text/email them when you need their support?
- Do you need to start putting out your running or walking clothes so you can head out straight away when you get home rather than heading for the pantry?
- Do you need to buy a book to write your thoughts in?

Again, what you need to do or steps you need to put in place will be very specific to the bumps or triggers you have identified – do take the time to think this through.

YOU TIME: Making your environment supportive of change

For your specific situations, what do you need to do to make sure that your environment supports change? Fill in your ideas in column **F. Making your environment supportive of change** of your own table.

REALITY CHECK

Please be aware that these changes will not happen overnight! Changing the way you think and your default habits and behaviours will take time and practice. I would encourage you to tackle one of your bumps and triggers at a time. You may need to refine your new thought and you may need to come up with three or four ideas for new things to do until you find a solution that works for you. The biggest thing is not to give up and not to judge yourself if you go back to your old ways sometimes. That, again, is NORMAL. What you are trying to achieve here is that, over time, you will choose your new thoughts and behaviours more often than your old ones. Eventually, you will hardly ever, and maybe never, think and do what you used to. But please be kind to yourself and be patient – miracles can happen, but not overnight.

As well as all these solutions, it is also important to note that if there are reasons why you are arguing with people, struggling at work or feeling lonely or depressed, you don't have to put up with these things if they are getting in the way of you living the life you really want and deserve. I have found the approach I am advising here to be very successful and it can work for you. However, if by doing this work on yourself you have raised some deep emotional issues which you just can't come to terms with, please, for goodness' sake, seek professional help. There are some superb psychologists and coaches out there who can help you work through this stuff on an individual level, which is really very important.

Bringing it all together

Hurray, you've made it! I hope you have enjoyed the journey of self-discovery along with what you have learnt about food and nutrition. I hope this book has given you the inspiration and ideas you need to change the way you eat and get the results you are looking for in your life, now and in the long term.

I have asked you to do a lot of work in this book and no doubt you will have a monster list of things to work on, but don't panic. Remember this is a journey and you are just at the beginning – it's exciting that there is so much to do!

There will be so many things from this book that you can take away and work on: meal planning, new recipe ideas, increasing your awareness when you are eating, reducing your portion sizes, label reading; and the list goes on. Do not be overwhelmed though, this really is a journey and to get permanent results, it will take time. I know that it is not as glam or sexy as detoxing or doing a six-week challenge that has a bikini model fronting the advertisement – but, as you know by now, the reason why I have written this book is because for 95 per cent of people those things don't work in the long term. I am guessing, if you're reading this now, they haven't worked for you.

This book is designed to help you change, step by step. Start with the basics: the meal planning, getting your recipes together. Once you have nailed that, move on to reading labels and taking time to get familiar with that side of food. From there, work on the habits, behaviours and challenges which are holding you back, one at a time. You will get there if you believe in yourself. Be assured, there will be ups and downs along the way, but it is totally, TOTALLY worth it – and so are you.

Let's just recap on a few things to make sure you can apply what you have learnt from today on:

- Take a look at your vision and goals again. Get a clear picture in your mind of how you want your life to be. Review your vision and goals every few months and alter them as needed.
- Be sure to sort out your personalised nutrition planner – this will help you establish a routine.
- ALWAYS plan your meals – always, every single week without fail, wherever you are.
- Identify times when you struggle to eat well, work out why that is and come up with some solutions.

- Cook smarter every day and use the healthy habits suggested in this book.
- Shop smarter, practise reading labels and make the best choice with each food group.
- If you don't already, why not try growing your own fruit and veggies?
- Always be mindful of your portions – use smaller plates, bowls and cutlery.
- Adapt your environment at home and at work to help you reach your goals.
- Keep up your hydration.
- Be mindful of unhelpful habits you may have with caffeinated drinks and alcohol.
- Try at least one new recipe a week.
- Aim to do a combination of cardiovascular, resistance and flexibility training every week.
- Create an exercise routine and get your friends and family involved, too.
- Take action on managing emotional eating and eating or drinking for the wrong reason.

Best of luck to you. Let me know how you get on and keep healthy and happy.

Claire

www.claireturnbull.co.nz

4

Can't-fail Quick-and-easy Recipes

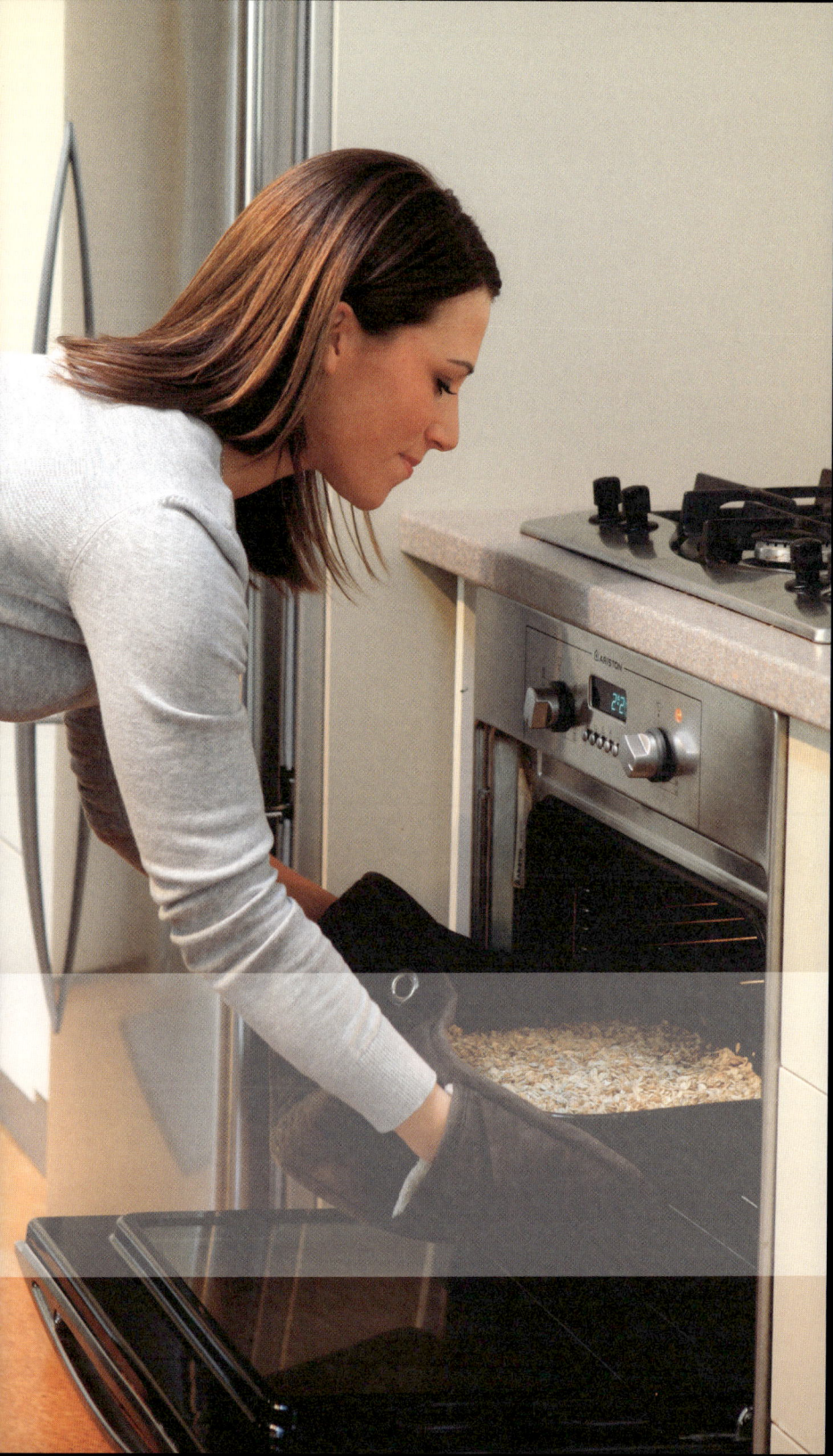

What is a healthy recipe?

The definition of a healthy recipe seems to vary dramatically depending on who you talk to. To some it will mean using all natural, home-grown ingredients. To others it's simply a meal which is served with vegetables. In my view a healthy recipe is one which is suitable for everyday eating, ideally made with fresh ingredients and providing a nice balance of nutrients as well as having an appropriate amount of energy (kJ) in the portion you intend to eat. I have put together some of my favourite everyday healthy recipes to provide you with some inspiration in the kitchen – I really hope you enjoy them!

BRILLIANT BREAKFASTS

A nutrient-packed breakfast is such an important start to the day! A good breakfast will provide you with the energy you need to get up and going as well as a good dose of vitamins, minerals and other nutritious goodies.

Brilliant breakfasts will include some combination of whole grains, low-fat dairy, a small amount of healthy fat as well as some fruit and/or vegetables. Here are my top picks for a healthy start to the day. They are all super delicious – I know you will love them.

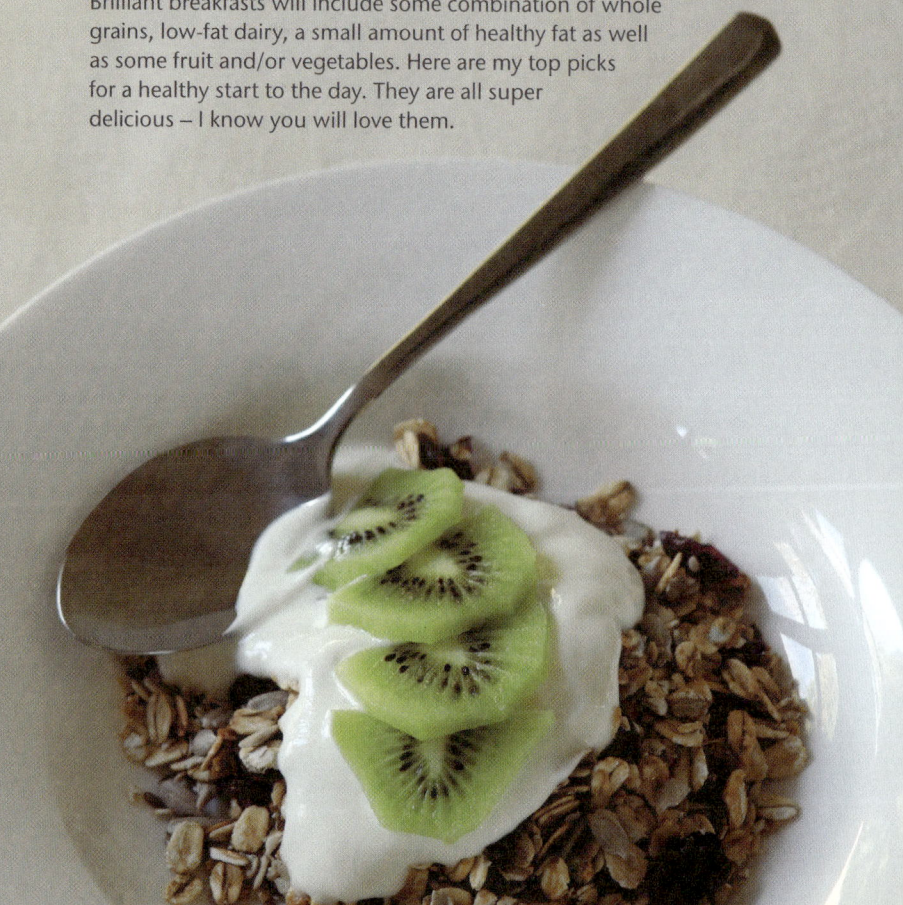

Mum's home-made muesli *(66 serves)*

My mum has made her own muesli for as long as I can remember. It's such a great thing to do. I really enjoy making my own cereal because I can use any ingredients I like and make it slightly different each time. You can use any combination of grains, nuts, seeds and dried fruits. Here is one of my favourite mixtures. This makes a large amount for everyone in my house but you can easily adapt the quantities and make less.

10 cups (about 1 kg) wholegrain oats

5 cups (about 500 g) rolled oats

2 cups rye flakes – alternatively add extra oats

¾ cup runny honey

1 cup pumpkin seeds

1 cup sunflower seeds

½ cup sesame seeds

½ cup linseeds

1 cup sultanas

1 cup dried cranberries

Preheat oven to 180 °C. Place wholegrain and rolled oats and rye into a large roasting tin.

Heat honey either in a saucepan on the stovetop or in a glass bowl or jug in the microwave for 10–15 seconds on high, until it is an easy pouring consistency.

Pour honey over oats and rye and stir through to get a light coating of honey on as many of the grains as possible.

Cook in the oven for about 10 minutes or until the grains start to turn slightly golden. Carefully remove the dish from the oven and stir grains with a large spoon. Place back in the oven for another 5–10 minutes. Remove again and stir. Repeat this process 3–4 times or until oats and rye are golden or browned to your liking.

Cool in the dish. When completely cool, stir through seeds and dried fruit. Store in an air-tight container.

Serve it up!
- Measure about ⅓ of a cup of muesli into a bowl and serve with ice-cold low-fat milk and/or 1–2 tablespoons of low-fat yoghurt. Yum!

Adapt it
- Replace some of the oats with barley flakes.
- Add chopped dried apricots instead of the cranberries.

Nutrition information in a ⅓ cup serving (without toppings)				
kJ = 757	Carbs = 29 g	Protein = 6 g	Fat = 5 g	Fibre = 4 g

Bircher muesli *(Serves 1)*

Looking for a healthy, filling, nutrient-packed breakfast? Bircher muesli is the answer. The added bonus is that it is incredibly economical and you can make so many different varieties depending on what you like.

My Bircher muesli is simply oats soaked in fruit juice, water or milk. You then add any combo of fruit, nuts and seeds – it's so delicious.

Another great thing about Bircher muesli is that you can also enjoy it at other times of the day. I often have a portion with low-fat yoghurt for my afternoon tea if I plan to head to the gym or for a run after work. I just make it in a small plastic container and keep it in the fridge at the office. It gives me the fuel I need to power through the training session and is far healthier than many other snacks.

½ cup oats
¼ cup apple juice
¼ cup water

Place oats in a bowl or plastic container with a lid. Pour over apple juice and water.

Cover and leave to soak for at least an hour (or overnight in the fridge if possible).

Eat and enjoy!

Serve it up!
- You can enjoy Bircher muesli on its own or make it more interesting by topping it with a large dollop of low-fat vanilla yoghurt (or unsweetened yoghurt with vanilla extract added) and a few walnuts, or with low-fat vanilla yoghurt and grated apple and, if you like, a pinch of cinnamon.

Adapt it
- For a sweeter Bircher muesli, use ½ cup of apple juice and no water.
- Soak in ½ cup of low-fat milk instead of apple juice.
- Try adding dried fruit, nuts and seeds, either before or after soaking. Some great combos are walnuts and dried cranberries or sliced almonds and sultanas.

Nutrition information per serve (without toppings)				
kJ = 727	Carbs = 33 g	Protein = 6 g	Fat = 2 g	Fibre = 4 g

Quick and easy porridge *(Serves 1)*

Time to go back to basics. Porridge makes a fantastic breakfast, particularly on a cold winter's morning. Here is the base recipe and my ideas for toppings.

½ cup oats
¼ cup water
⅓ cup low-fat milk

Tip
- Add more or less water depending on how thick or thin you like your porridge.

Stovetop method
Place oats, water and milk into a non-stick saucepan. Cook over a medium heat for around 3–4 minutes or until thick and creamy – done!

Microwave method
Place oats, water and milk in to a deep microwave-proof bowl. Cook in the microwave on high for 1 minute, then take out and stir.

Place it back in the microwave for another minute, watching at all times to make sure it doesn't bubble over the bowl, then take out and stir. Depending on the type of oats you use and how powerful your microwave is, it may now be done or need another minute or so to finish cooking.

Serve it up!
- Top with a few sultanas or currants for natural sweetness and a splash of cold milk if you like.

Adapt it
- Stir through 2 teaspoons of ground LSA (linseeds, sunflower seeds and almonds) and drizzle with a teaspoon of honey.
- When porridge has cooked for 2 minutes, throw in a small handful of frozen berries and cook for the remaining time – a delicious, healthy addition.
- When the porridge is cooked, stir in a scoop of vanilla or chocolate protein powder for a protein-packed breakfast.
- Add a small pinch of either cinnamon and/or mixed spice at the start to make a delicious spicy porridge.
- Top with a small sliced banana and a teaspoon of runny honey for a super-filling breakfast.

Nutrition information per serve (without toppings)				
kJ = 737	Carbs = 29 g	Protein = 9 g	Fat = 3 g	Fibre = 4 g

Oaty nut mix with yoghurt and fruit *(36 serves)*

This is by far one of my all-time favourite breakfasts. I have it with low-fat unsweetened yoghurt with some kind of fresh or stewed fruit on top and a tablespoon of the oaty mix for a topping – it is just so good!

4 cups rolled oats
2 cups oat bran
2 cups ground LSA
1 cup walnuts,
    chopped
6 tsp cinnamon or
    mixed spice

Mix everything together and store in a sealed airtight container in the fridge.

Serve it up!
- Serve a ¼ cup of oaty nut mix with 150 g of unsweetened natural yoghurt and 4 tablespoons of either stewed apple, rhubarb, plums, berries or a grated apple or pear.

Adapt it
- Swap the walnuts for almonds, hazelnuts or sunflower seeds.

Tip
- To make sure nuts stay fresh, they are best stored in the fridge!

Nutrition information per serve (with toppings)				
kJ = 802	Carbs = 21 g	Protein = 11 g	Fat = 6 g	Fibre = 4 g

Mighty cook-up *(Serves 1)*

Let's be honest, most cooked breakfasts get a bad name. Some of them are indeed SHOCKING, with more kilojoules and fat than you need in a whole day served up on the one plate. But, the great news is that you can have a healthy cooked breakfast. Here is my favourite version.

oil – in a spray bottle
1 tomato, halved
2 fresh eggs – ideally free range
1 slice grainy bread
2 handfuls of baby spinach
2 thin slices of avocado
ground black pepper

Heat a few sprays of oil in a non-stick frying pan. Add tomato halves skin side down and cook for 1 minute. Turn tomato over and brown for another minute or so.

Meanwhile, fill a second frying pan or shallow saucepan with 3 cm of boiling water. Put the pan on a medium heat and heat until very small bubbles appear in the water (not too many, though).

Crack eggs into the water and poach for about 1 minute or to your liking. While eggs are poaching, put toast on.

Place spinach in a microwave-proof bowl and cook on high (no water needed) for 30 seconds to allow it to soften.

When the eggs are cooked, remove from the water with a slotted spoon, allowing all the water to drain.

Place eggs on toast and serve with sliced avocado, tomato and spinach. Season with pepper – yum!

Adapt it
- Why not have some mushrooms, too? You can fry them with the tomato and season with lots of freshly ground black pepper.
- Try spinach mixed with silverbeet and kale for mixed greeny goodness.

Tip
- Remember, as good as avocado is for you, it is high in kilojoules so be mindful of your portions.

Nutrition information per serve				
kJ = 1327	Carbs = 22 g	Protein = 20 g	Fat = 17 g	Fibre = 6 g

Omelette with spinach and salmon (Serves 1)

Omelettes are excellent for breakfast, but are a great lunch option, too. They can also make a quick and easy dinner when things are busy and time is short. Omelettes are packed with protein and make it easy to get in a few servings of veggies as part of your meal.

2 eggs – ideally free
    range
2 tbsp water
ground black pepper
chopped fresh
    chives, optional
oil – in a spray bottle
handful of baby
    spinach
6 cherry tomatoes,
    cut in half
50 g smoked salmon

Beat eggs and water together in a small bowl. Season with pepper and add chopped chives if using.

Heat a small non-stick frying pan and spray with a few pumps of oil. Pour eggs into the frying pan and tilt the pan forwards, backwards, left and right until the liquid egg covers the whole base of the pan.

Cook for 30 seconds to 1 minute or until the edges start to firm up. As the edges start to firm slightly, tilt the pan and use a small spatula to draw the cooked edge of the omelette into the centre. The liquid egg will flow into the space. Repeat until no liquid egg remains. Top with spinach, tomatoes and salmon.

When the egg is looking firm, fold in half and cook for another 30 seconds or so, depending on how well cooked you like your omelette.

Serve it up!
- Simply slip the omelette onto a plate, top with a handful of fresh baby spinach or rocket, if you like, then eat and enjoy.

Adapt it
- Use finely chopped red onion, tomato and mushrooms.

Tips
- Avoid overbeating the eggs; if you whip them to death you can end up with a rubbery omelette.
- If you prefer your veggies cooked a little more, soften them in a frying pan with a little oil before you start, then add to the part-cooked omelette.

Nutrition information per serve				
kJ = 1084	Carbs = 3 g	Protein = 25 g	Fat = 16 g	Fibre = 2 g

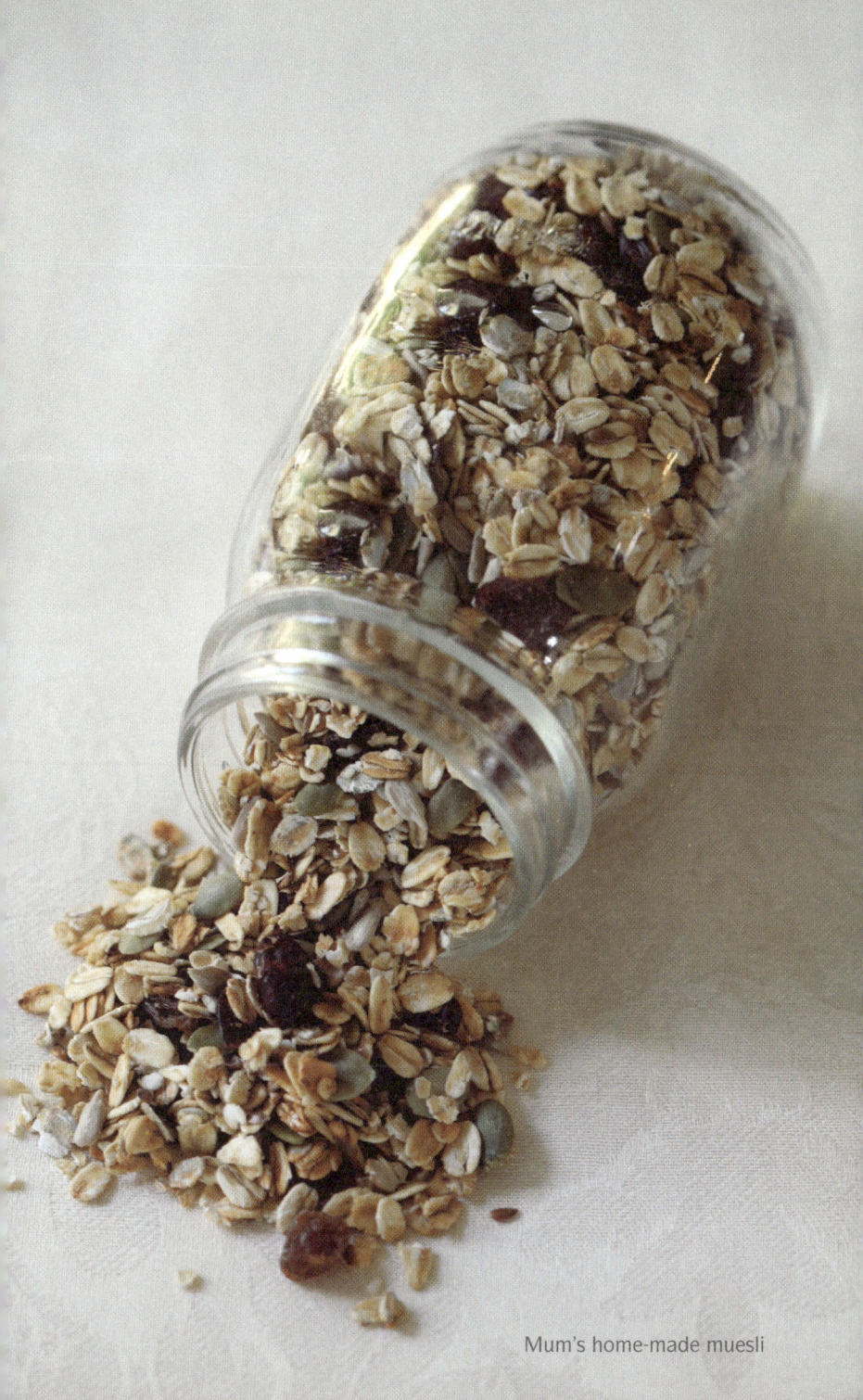

Mum's home-made muesli

SMOOTHIES

I am just the biggest smoothie fan. You can make so many delicious flavour combinations and they make such a great breakfast or light lunch at the weekend – particularly if you have started the day with a cooked breakfast.

Smoothies are an easy way to get a fruit serve, one or two dairy serves and some healthy fat as well. You can also add certain vegetables to smoothies (mainly spinach) and get a veggie serve, too! Here are some of my best smoothie combos. Simply put all the ingredients for each recipe into a blender and blitz or put the ingredients into a jug and use a stick blender to combine everything. You can add extra milk or water if you prefer a thinner consistency.

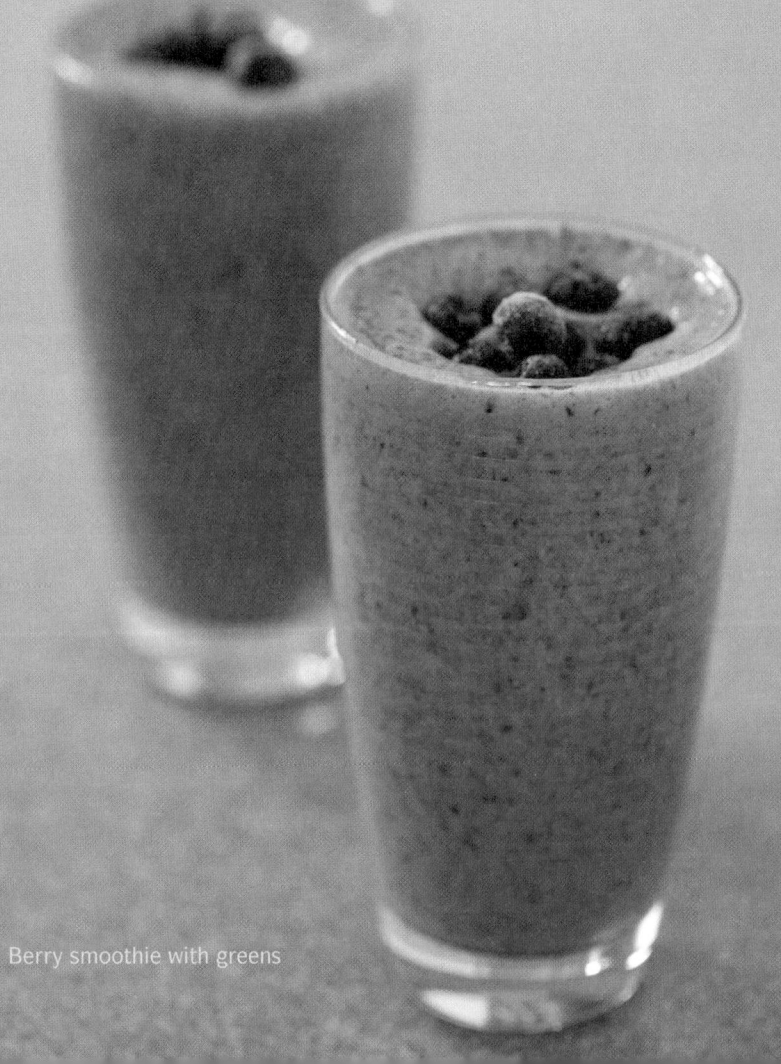

Berry smoothie with greens

Berry smoothie with greens

100 ml trim milk
100 ml water – add more if needed
2 tbsp vanilla or chocolate protein powder
1/2 cup blueberries
handful of baby spinach
1 tsp cinnamon
2 tsp ground LSA
3–4 big ice cubes

Nutrition information per serve				
kJ = 830	Carbs = 22 g	Protein = 19 g	Fat = 4 g	Fibre = 4 g

Banana and oat thick-shake

200 ml trim milk
2 tbsp low-fat unsweetened or vanilla yoghurt
1 small banana
1 heaped tbsp rolled oats
1 tsp runny honey

Nutrition information per serve				
kJ = 1019	Carbs = 45 g	Protein = 13 g	Fat = 2 g	Fibre = 2 g

Peach and strawberry smoothie

1 large fresh peach, skin removed, or 2–3 peach halves from a can
150 ml trim milk
3 tbsp low-fat strawberry or berry yoghurt
2 tsp ground LSA

Tips
- LSA is a mixture of ground linseeds, sunflower seeds and almonds – you can make your own or pick it up from a health food store or supermarket.
- Use soy milk, rice milk or lactose-free milk.

Nutrition information per serve				
kJ = 589	Carbs = 18 g	Protein = 10 g	Fat = 3 g	Fibre = 2 g

LIVELY LUNCHES

Some people don't mind eating the same thing for lunch day-in and day-out, but, personally, I have to mix things up. I always like to have something to look forward to when it comes to my lunch, as well as knowing that what I eat will be ideal nourishment for my body and mind!

Recap: an ideal balanced lunch is:

- 1–2 servings of veggies
- 1 serving of meat/fish or a protein alternative
- Some healthy starch
- Small amount of healthy fat.

SALADS

First up, we have some fabulous salad recipes which I just love for lunch. You can often make these using leftovers from your evening meal if you plan ahead. Don't be afraid to mix and match ingredients to make your own versions of these salads!

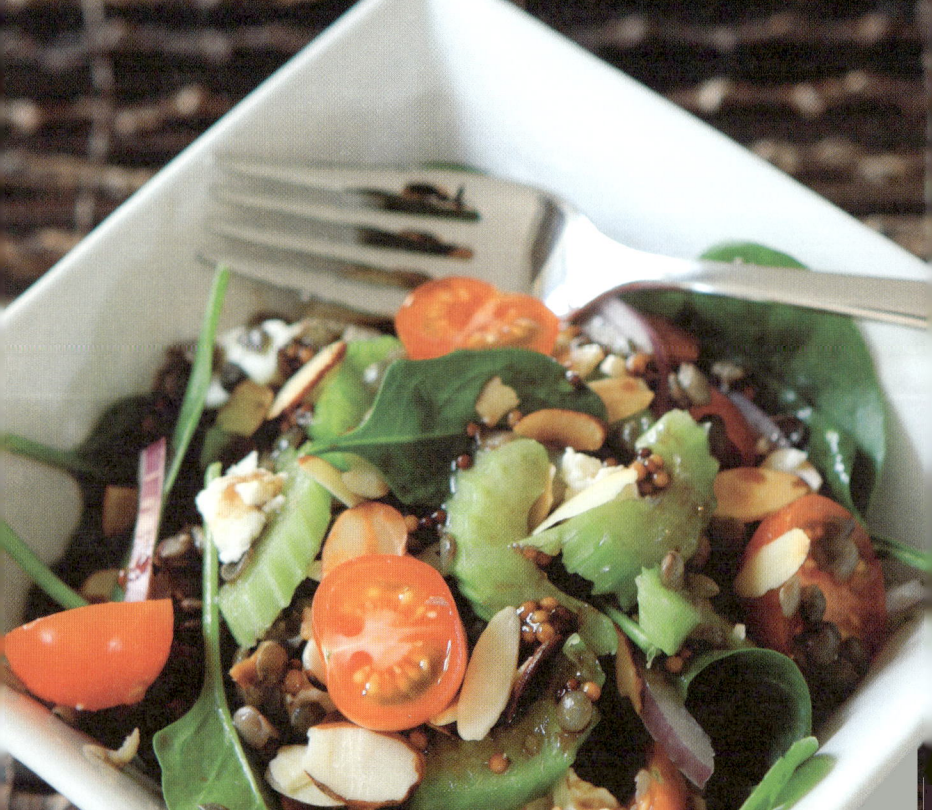

Spinach, lentil and celery salad *(Serves 2)*

This is a colourful salad which is great for lunch any day of the week.

½ cup Puy lentils
   (French green
   lentils)
2 cups boiling water
oil – in a spray bottle
20 g sliced almonds
2–3 large handfuls
   of baby spinach
2 sticks of celery,
   thinly sliced on
   the diagonal
1 small red onion,
   very finely sliced
8 cherry tomatoes,
   cut in half
30 g goat's feta
   cheese

Balsamic dressing
2 tsp olive oil
2 tbsp balsamic
   vinegar
1 heaped tsp honey
1 tsp wholegrain
   mustard
ground black pepper

Wash lentils in a sieve until the water runs clear. Place in a saucepan with boiling water and boil for 15–20 minutes or until lentils are soft and tender but not mushy. Drain and rinse with cold water. Set aside.

Heat a non-stick frying pan, spray with a few pumps of oil and add sliced almonds. Toast for a minute until light golden brown – be sure not to burn them! Remove from the heat and set aside.

Mix remaining salad ingredients together in a large bowl.

Mix all ingredients for the dressing together in a small jug and pour over the salad. Toss gently to combine.

Serve it up!
• Divide the salad between two plates and enjoy.

Adapt it
• Add lemon juice as a dressing rather than the balsamic dressing.

Nutrition information per serve (without dressing)				
kJ = 1301	Carbs = 35 g	Protein = 19 g	Fat = 11 g	Fibre = 18 g

Nutrition information per serve (with dressing)				
kJ = 1537	Carbs = 39 g	Protein = 19 g	Fat = 15 g	Fibre = 18 g

Spinach and pumpkin salad *(Serves 2)*

This is a satisfying, flavour-packed salad which is SO easy to make.

¼ (about 300 g) small pumpkin, chopped into cubes
oil – in a spray bottle
salt and ground black pepper
1 tsp ground cumin
2 large handfuls of baby spinach
2 sticks of celery, thinly sliced on the diagonal
30 g goat's cheese, chopped into small cubes
8 walnuts, chopped in half

Preheat oven to 180 °C. Line a baking tray with baking paper.

Place chopped pumpkin on the prepared tray. Spray with a few pumps of oil and season with a small amount of salt and pepper. Sprinkle with cumin.

Bake for 15–20 minutes or until pumpkin is soft. Remove from the oven and cool.

Place the cooled pumpkin into a bowl with the rest of the ingredients and mix together.

Serve it up!
- Divide the salad between two plates (or one plate and a plastic container to have for lunch the next day) and enjoy.
- To make this a nutritionally balanced lunch you need to add some additional protein. Try serving the salad with a chopped boiled egg or a small can of tuna.
- You can add a squeeze of fresh lemon or balsamic vinegar to liven things up, too! If you are taking this to work, put a wedge of lemon into your lunchbox and squeeze over just before eating.

Nutrition information per serve (without boiled egg)				
kJ = 962	Carbs = 8 g	Protein = 10 g	Fat = 18 g	Fibre = 4 g

Nutrition information per serve (with boiled egg)				
kJ = 1275	Carbs = 8 g	Protein = 16 g	Fat = 23 g	Fibre = 4 g

Delicious carrot and currant salad *(Serves 4)*

When we think salad, lettuce is often the first thing that springs to mind, but this gorgeous, crunchy salad is oh so different. Using carrots as the base, it is just delicious!

oil – in a spray bottle
¼ cup sliced
   almonds
4 large carrots,
   peeled and grated
2 sticks of celery,
   thinly sliced on
   the diagonal
½ cup grated tasty
   or edam cheese
1 can (390 g) butter
   beans, washed
   and drained – or
   cooked yourself!
½ cup currants
handful of finely
   chopped parsley

Heat a non-stick frying pan, spray with a few pumps of oil and add sliced almonds. Toast for a minute until light golden brown – be sure not to burn them! Remove from the heat.

Mix all ingredients together – it is now ready to serve.

Serve it up!
- To make this a nutritionally balanced meal, add some protein. Cooked shredded chicken is ideal in this salad, or it is also great served with steak, lamb or fish.

Adapt it
- Instead of butter beans, try chickpeas. You can try cooking the butter beans or chickpeas yourself rather than using canned.

Nutrition information per serve (without meat or fish)				
kJ = 1051	Carbs = 17 g	Protein = 13 g	Fat = 14 g	Fibre = 5 g

Red cabbage salad *(Serves 4)*

This is my mum's recipe and I make it all the time – it is so easy and incredibly tasty, always a winner!

½ red cabbage,
    finely shredded
2 large carrots,
    peeled and grated
1 large eating apple,
    skin on, grated
½ cup raisins
3 tbsp lite salad
    dressing
3 tsp ground
    coriander
handful of chopped
    fresh coriander

Mix everything together and it is done.

Serve it up!
• To make this a nutritionally balanced meal, add some protein. This is fabulous served with fish, chicken or any grilled lean meat.
• If you plan to take the salad for lunch, have it with a boiled egg, or canned tuna, salmon or sardines or some cold lean meat. For vegetarians, add some chickpeas, butter beans or kidney beans and a few nuts.

Adapt it
• Use currants or sultanas instead of raisins.
• Instead of the lite salad dressing, use 3 tbsp of lite sour cream and a squeeze of lemon juice.
• Add a can of chickpeas if you want a more filling salad.

Nutrition information per serve (without added protein)				
kJ = 472	Carbs = 22 g	Protein = 3 g	Fat = 1 g	Fibre = 7 g

Mango chicken salad *(Serves 4)*

This is a recipe my mother-in-law regularly makes for lunch.
It's super tasty.

1 large fresh mango,
   peeled (or 1 x
   425 g can sliced
   mango, drained)
300 g cooked and
   shredded chicken
1 tbsp mango
   chutney
4 large handfuls of
   salad greens (I like
   soft fancy lettuce
   for this salad)
handful of red or
   green grapes
½ small avocado,
   cut into chunks

Chop mango into small strips. Mix with shredded chicken and mango chutney.

Roughly tear lettuce and place on a serving dish.

Scatter chicken and mango mixture, grapes and avocado on top.

Serve it up!

- Enjoy this salad with a slice of grainy bread or a few grainy crackers if you need starch at lunchtime. Or just add some chickpeas or leftover roasted veggies such as kumara and potato.

Nutrition information per serve (without extra starch)				
kJ = 934	Carbs = 15 g	Protein = 25 g	Fat = 7 g	Fibre = 3 g

Chicken, corn and chickpea salad *(Serves 4)*

This is one of the quickest, easiest throw-together lunches that I know –
you can't go wrong with this!

400 g cooked and
shredded chicken
1½ cups (250 g)
cooked chickpeas
(or 1 x 400 g
can chickpeas,
drained)
1½ cups frozen corn,
defrosted (or 1 x
400 g can sweet-
corn, drained)
1 bag (120 g) baby
spinach or salad
greens
½ avocado, chopped
chopped fresh
coriander

Mix all ingredients together in a bowl – it is
that easy.

Serve it up!
• Serve with a squeeze of lemon juice or sweet chilli sauce for variety and
extra flavour.

Adapt it
• When corn is in season, use fresh instead of frozen or canned.

Tip
• 250 g chickpeas is the weight of a 400 g can which has been drained.

Nutrition information per serve (without chilli sauce)				
kJ = 1505	Carbs = 24 g	Protein = 38 g	Fat = 12 g	Fibre = 10 g

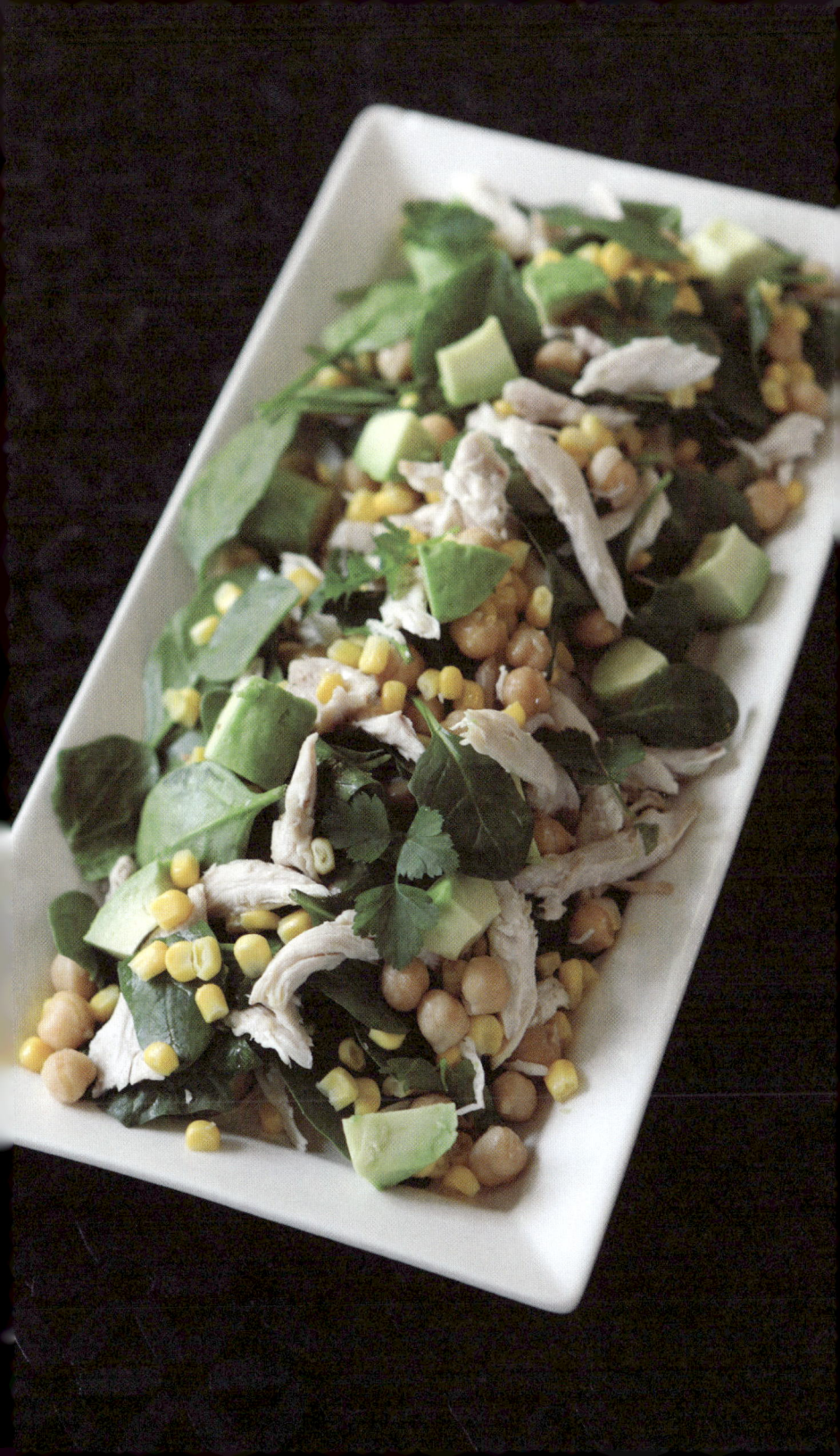

Tuna Niçoise *(Serves 2)*

This is one of my all-time favourite salads and my husband is a big fan, too. We grow our own cos lettuce (it is so easy – you must try it!) and we regularly enjoy this salad for weekend lunch in summer.

4 egg-sized potatoes
2 boiled eggs
180 g can tuna in spring water, drained
1 tbsp lite mayonnaise
juice of ½ a lemon
1 tsp capers, chopped
1–2 anchovies, very finely chopped
10 black olives, sliced in half
6 cherry tomatoes, sliced in half
3 cups shredded cos lettuce
1 tbsp grated Parmesan

Peel potatoes and boil in water until cooked, around 15 minutes. Drain and set aside to cool. Meanwhile, boil eggs, de-shell and chop into quarters. Set to one side.

Combine tuna, mayonnaise, lemon juice, capers and anchovies in a large bowl.

Add olives, tomatoes and lettuce. Mix together until well combined.

Serve with chopped potatoes, eggs and a sprinkling of grated Parmesan.

Nutrition information per serve

kJ = 1740	Carbs = 40 g	Protein = 39 g	Fat = 11 g	Fibre = 7 g

Crunchy coleslaw *(Serves 4)*

This is a brilliant base for a healthy lunch. You can make enough to last two or three days, which is fantastic. I serve this coleslaw with tuna, salmon, chicken or a boiled egg. You can also add a can of chickpeas or butter beans for a more filling option.

½ white cabbage, very finely sliced
2 large carrots, peeled and grated
1 small red onion, very finely chopped
handful of finely chopped mint and parsley
1 red chilli, very finely chopped, optional

Mix all ingredients together and store in the fridge in a plastic container. Store for 2–3 days.

Serve it up!
- Best to add the dressing, if using (see variations below), just before you eat it, so the whole batch doesn't go soggy.

Adapt it
- Make a quick dressing for the coleslaw from 1 teaspoon of lite mayonnaise, 1 teaspoon of lite sour cream, 1 tablespoon of water or lemon juice and freshly ground black pepper.
- Alternatively, a balsamic dressing would work well (see Spinach, lentil and celery salad on page 229).

Nutrition information per serve (without dressing)				
kJ = 165	Carbs = 7 g	Protein = 3 g	Fat = <1 g	Fibre = 4 g

SOUPS

Soup makes a great lunch in the winter months. It is also a good idea to have some soup in the fridge and/or freezer on standby for a quick, filling and healthy snack.

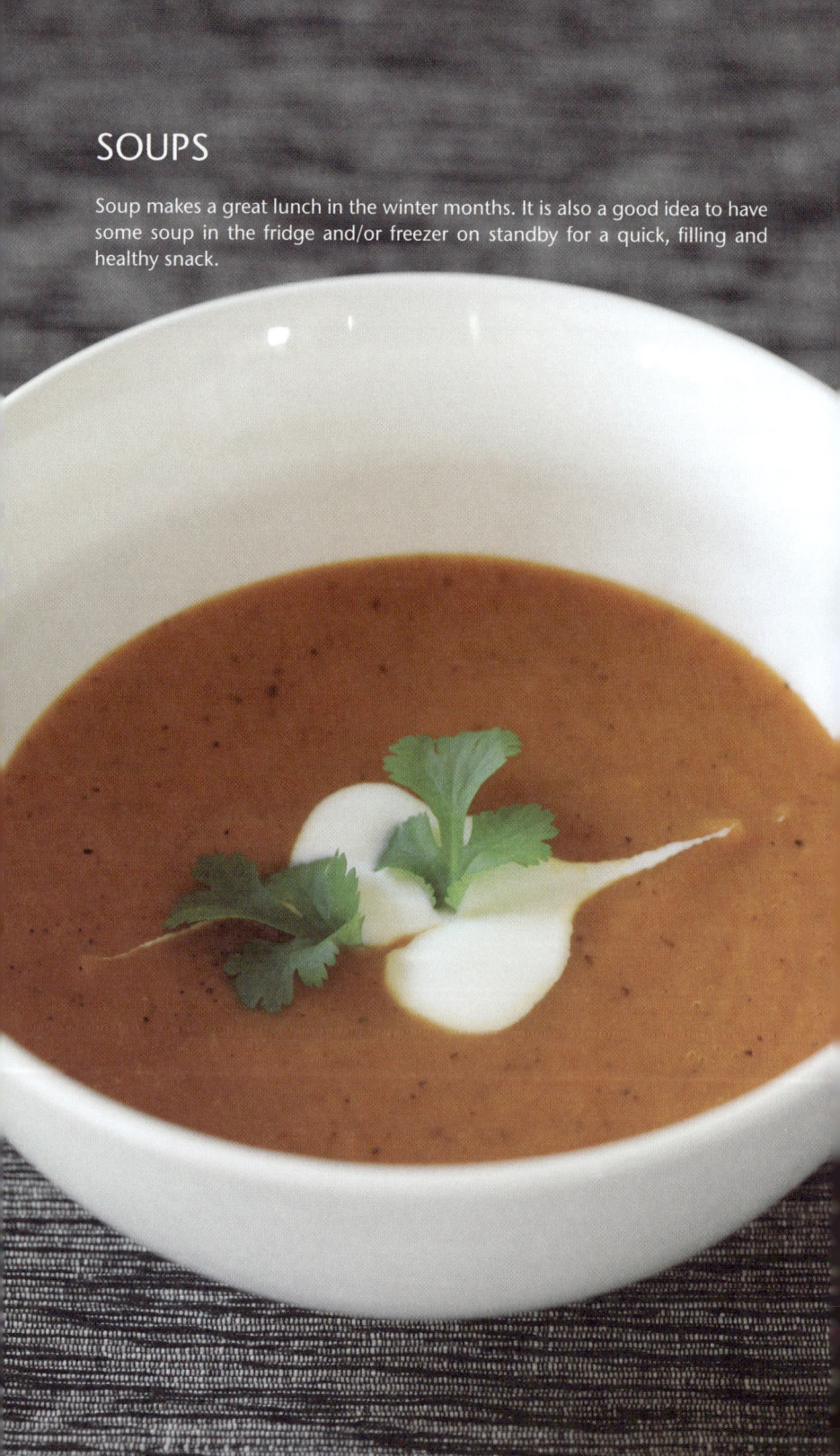

Carrot and coriander soup *(Serves 4–6)*

This is a British classic (and my mum's favourite) which you just have to try. It tastes even better when you make it with your own home-grown carrots.

1 tbsp coriander
   seeds
2 tsp oil
1 kg carrots, peeled
   and chopped
1 small clove garlic,
   crushed
1½ litres (6 cups)
   chicken or
   vegetable stock
   – home-made if
   possible

Dry-roast coriander seeds in a small frying pan over a medium heat for 1–2 minutes. Transfer to a mortar and pestle and crush.

In a large saucepan or stockpot, heat oil. Add carrots, garlic and crushed coriander seeds and cook on a low heat for 5–10 minutes.

Add stock and bring to the boil. Reduce the heat and simmer for 15–20 minutes until carrot is soft.

Remove from the heat and blend with a stick blender or in a blender – do this in several batches if necessary.

Serve it up!
• Serve with a small dollop of lite sour cream and fresh coriander.

Nutrition information per serve (without lite sour cream)				
kJ = 369	Carbs = 10 g	Protein = 5 g	Fat = 3 g	Fibre = 8 g

Nutrition information per serve (with lite sour cream)				
kJ = 410	Carbs = 10 g	Protein = 5 g	Fat = 4 g	Fibre = 8 g

Leek and cauliflower soup *(Serves 4)*

This is the easiest soup recipe you will ever find and the bonus is that it tastes SO good!

2 tsp oil
3 leeks, sliced
2 cloves garlic, crushed
1 large cauliflower, chopped into large florets
1½ litres (6 cups) vegetable or chicken stock – ideally home-made

Heat oil in a large saucepan or stockpot, then add leeks and garlic. Cook over a medium heat until soft.

Add cauliflower and stock. Cover and bring to the boil.

Reduce heat to a simmer and cook for 15–20 minutes or until cauliflower is very soft.

Blend in a blender – do this in batches if necessary – or with a stick blender.

Serve it up!

• Serve with a small dollop of lite sour cream or natural yoghurt and freshly chopped parsley.

Nutrition information per serve (without lite sour cream)				
kJ = 417	Carbs = 10 g	Protein = 8 g	Fat = 3 g	Fibre = 6 g

Nutrition information per serve (with lite sour cream)				
kJ = 457	Carbs = 10 g	Protein = 8 g	Fat = 4 g	Fibre = 6 g

Thick curried lentil soup *(Serves 4)*

If you enjoy a soup packed full of flavour, then look no further!

1 cup red lentils,
  rinsed
few chunky slices
  of fresh ginger
2 bay leaves
3 cups water
1 tsp oil
1 onion, finely
  chopped
2 cloves garlic,
  crushed
2 tsp ground
  turmeric
1 tsp ground cumin
1/2 tsp garam masala
1/2 tsp chilli flakes
2 tbsp lemon juice
1/2–1 tsp iodised salt
2–3 cups boiling
  water

In a large saucepan place lentils, ginger, bay leaves and water and bring to the boil.

Reduce the heat to a simmer and cook for 10 minutes. Stir to prevent sticking. Remove ginger and bay leaves. Set lentils aside.

Heat oil in a frying pan over a medium heat. Add onion and cook for 3 minutes.

Stir in garlic, spices and chilli flakes, and cook for a further minute.

Add onion mixture to lentils and stir well. Place back on the heat and cook for a few more minutes. Keep stirring.

Stir in lemon juice and salt.

Add extra boiling water (you are likely to need a few cups) to make the soup a consistency of your liking.

Adapt it

• You can use 2–3 teaspoons of curry paste rather than the spices to make the cooking time quicker if you are in a rush.

Nutrition information per serve				
kJ = 728	Carbs = 26 g	Protein = 12 g	Fat = 2 g	Fibre = 5 g

MAIN MEALS

For a healthy balanced dinner, aim to have half your plate full of non-starchy vegetables, a quarter protein-containing foods and no more than a quarter of starchy foods.

Some of the recipes in this section suggest that you serve the dish with rice, quinoa or pasta on the side as well as veggies or salad, of course.

Pages 252–3 show the nutrition information for different serving sizes of each of the various sides so you can work out how many kilojoules your overall meal is, based on the serving size you choose.

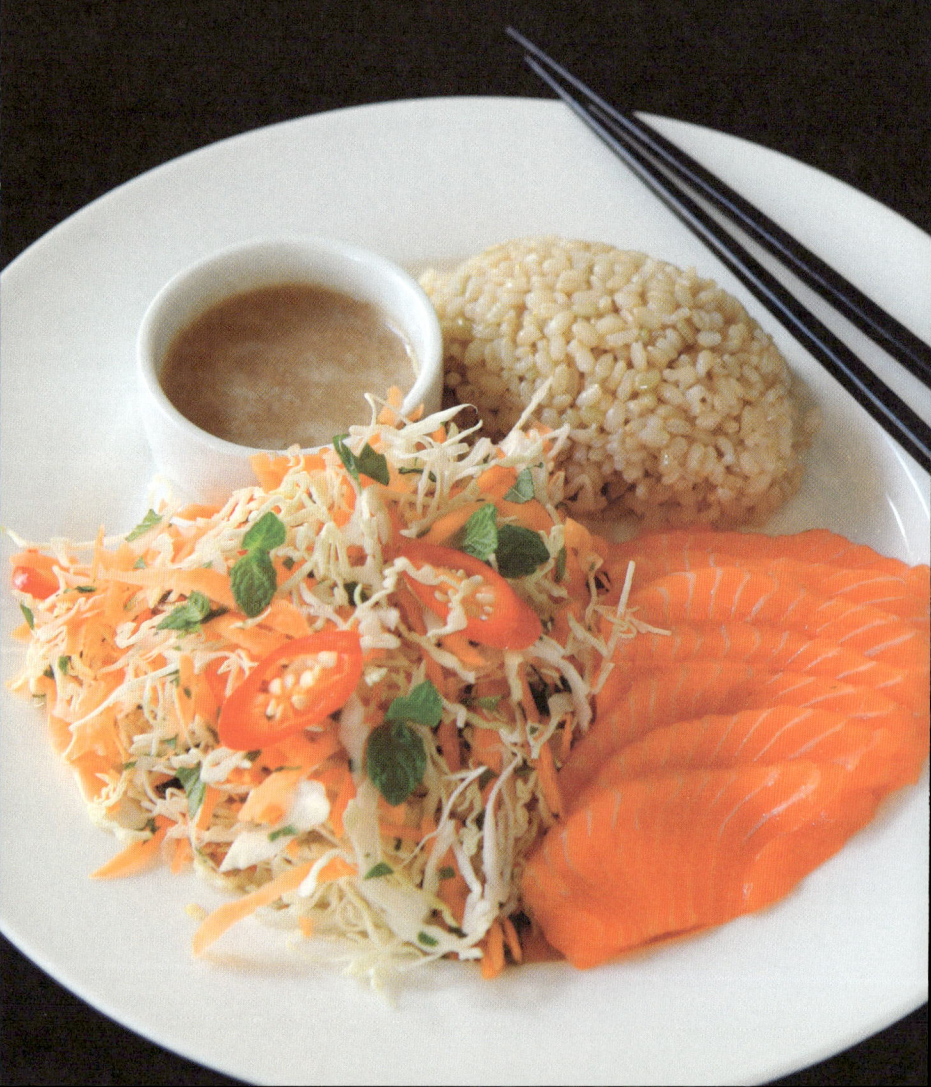

Salmon sashimi with coleslaw and brown rice *(Serves 4)*

I adore salmon and when you buy it fresh, it can be enjoyed raw sashimi style. This is a quick and easy dinner that I enjoy as often as I can – I am sure you will love it too!

1½ cups brown rice
3 cups water
½ quantity coleslaw, see page 237
400 g fresh New Zealand king salmon, very thinly sliced

Dressing
2 tsp oil
2 tsp sesame oil
2 tbsp vinegar – I use sushi vinegar but cider or white is fine
1 tbsp reduced-salt soy sauce
1 tbsp toasted sesame seeds
1 clove garlic, crushed
1 tbsp sugar dissolved in 3 tbsp water

Cook brown rice in water on the stovetop or in the microwave for around 25 minutes.

While the rice is cooking, make the dressing by putting all ingredients into a blender and blitzing for a minute. Alternatively, you can place the dressing ingredients into a screwtop jar and shake them together.

Divide cooked rice between 4 bowls. Place a handful of coleslaw on top and scatter with sliced salmon, or arrange on the plate as shown opposite.

Pour over dressing and you are ready to go!

Adapt it
• You can absolutely cook the salmon first if you prefer. The easiest way is to divide the 400 g into 4 portions, place on a tray lined with baking paper and pop into an oven preheated to 180 °C for 8–10 minutes or until cooked to your liking.

Nutrition information per serve (with rice and coleslaw)

kJ = 2260	Carbs = 62 g	Protein = 28 g	Fat = 20 g	Fibre = 5 g

Prawn, leek and garlic risotto *(Serves 6)*

Traditionally risottos are very high in fat, packed with butter and often cream too, as well as being light on vegetables. This is my healthy version. I have made this for my family and friends loads of times and the feedback is always brilliant!

2–3 large leeks
2 tsp oil
1 large onion, chopped
2 cloves garlic, crushed
1½ cups risotto rice (arborio)
4 cups chicken or vegetable stock – home-made or made from cubes
1 cup frozen peas
2 cups fresh spinach, chopped – or 1 cup frozen chopped spinach
400 g prawns, defrosted, deveined and rinsed
½ x 125 g tub extra lite cream cheese (such as light Philadelphia)
Parmesan to season

Prepare the leek by removing the tough green top and outer layer. Trim the bottom of the leek to remove any roots, then slice each leek in half lengthways and rinse well. Slice the leek finely.

Heat the oil in a large non-stick frying pan. Add onion, garlic and leeks. Cook over a medium heat until soft.

Add risotto rice and 1 cup of stock to the pan. Cook for 5 minutes, stirring every minute, until stock has evaporated.

Add remaining 3 cups of stock to the pan and cook for 15 minutes or until the rice is tender, stirring every few minutes.

Add peas and fresh or frozen spinach and cook for another 5 minutes.

Add prawns and cook for another 3–5 minutes or until prawns are cooked through.

Stir through lite cream cheese and add a splash of milk if needed to loosen the risotto. Sprinkle with a little Parmesan.

Serve it up!
• Serve with a large green salad.

Adapt it
• Make this risotto with chicken instead of prawns.
• For a special occasion, use 3 cups of stock with 1 cup of wine.

Nutrition information per serve (without green salad)				
kJ = 1370	Carbs = 49 g	Protein = 24 g	Fat = 4 g	Fibre = 5 g

Quick fish curry *(Serves 2)*

This is the perfect recipe to have at hand if you have had a really busy day and need a super-quick dinner.

1 tsp oil 1 onion, chopped	Heat oil in a non-stick frying pan and add onion. Cook for a few minutes until soft.
2 tsp curry paste – make your own if you have time!	Add curry paste and tomatoes, and bring to a simmer.
1 x 400 g can chopped tomatoes	Add fish fillets to the pan and cover in tomato curry sauce.
2 fish fillets (300 g for both), fresh or frozen	Put a lid on the pan and simmer for a few minutes until fish is cooked through.
2 tbsp lite sour cream	Just before serving, stir sour cream into the sauce to make it creamy.

Serve it up!
- Serve with rice and green veggies of your choice.

Adapt it
- Use Indian-flavoured tomatoes if you like.
- Add chopped chilli or chilli flakes if you like your food spicy.
- Make your own curry paste by heating 2 tsp garam masala, 2 tsp turmeric, 2 tsp ground cumin and 2 tsp ground coriander seeds for a few minutes. In a small blender place 1 sliced fresh chilli (or 1 tsp chilli powder – more if you like heat), 2 crushed garlic cloves, 1 tbsp freshly grated ginger, a pinch of iodised salt, 1 tbsp oil and 2 tbsp tomato paste. Add the spices to the blender and whizz it all together. This will be enough to make a few curries, so keep what you don't use in the fridge.

Tips
- If you are using frozen fish, ideally defrost it before cooking. However, if you forget you can absolutely cook the fish from frozen – just cook it for an additional 5 or so minutes until cooked through.
- If you have brown rice with this recipe, remember it takes a while to cook so put that on first and then start prepping everything for the curry – all going well, everything will then be ready at the same time.

Nutrition information per serve (without rice or green veggies)				
kJ = 1230	Carbs = 15 g	Protein = 34 g	Fat = 11 g	Fibre = 4 g

Super chilli *(Serves 4)*

Chilli is my one of my family's favourite meals, so I have learnt to make a really healthy version because if it's not on the menu there are complaints! I include red lentils to make the meat go further and to add some fibre – the great thing is that no one even knows they are in there.

$1/3$ cup red lentils
1 cup boiling water
1 tsp oil
1 onion, finely chopped
1 chilli, finely chopped
400 g lean beef mince
1 x 400 g can chopped tomatoes
2 tbsp tomato purée
$1^1/2$ cups cooked kidney beans (or 1 x 400 g can, drained and rinsed)

Rinse lentils in a sieve until the water runs clear. Place in a saucepan with boiling water and cook for about 10 minutes or until lentils are soft and all the water has been absorbed. Be sure to watch the pan carefully and keep stirring to prevent the lentils from sticking to the bottom. Remove from the heat and set aside.

Heat oil in a non-stick frying pan. Add onion and chilli, and cook for 2–3 minutes until soft.

Add mince to the pan and brown for 5 minutes.

Add tomatoes, tomato purée and kidney beans and bring to a simmer.

Add cooked red lentils to mince mixture and stir through. Cook for 10 minutes.

Serve it up!
• Serve with rice and lots of veggies.

Adapt it
• Use cooked black beans instead of or as well as the kidney beans – they are delicious.

Nutrition information per serve (without rice or veggies)				
kJ = 1021	Carbs = 14 g	Protein = 28 g	Fat = 8 g	Fibre = 4 g

Tandoori chicken *(Serves 4)*

This is a super-quick dinner which is always a winner in my house. I love this with a big green salad or coleslaw.

2 tbsp tandoori paste

4 tbsp unsweetened natural yoghurt

400 g skinless chicken breast or thighs, sliced into bite-sized pieces

Preheat oven to 180 °C. Line a tray with tin foil.

Place tandoori paste and yoghurt in a large bowl and mix together.

Add chicken slices to yoghurt mixture and stir through. Ideally leave to marinate for 1 hour in the fridge – but if you don't have time, not to worry.

Place yoghurt-coated chicken on the prepared tray.

Bake for 10 minutes or until chicken is cooked through.

Serve it up!
• Serve with brown or basmati rice and a mixed salad of your choice.

Adapt it
• Cook poppadoms for 1 minute in the microwave – a great addition to this meal.
• A teaspoon of mango chutney and lime pickle also adds an extra delicious touch.

Nutrition information per serve (without rice or salad)				
kJ = 783	Carbs = 1 g	Protein = 32 g	Fat = 6 g	Fibre = <1 g

Thai-style prawns with crunchy veggies
(Serves 4)

This is an impressive-looking salad which is very easy to prepare.

1 red capsicum,
    deseeded and
    thinly sliced
1 yellow capsicum,
    deseeded and
    thinly sliced
⅓ large cucumber,
    thinly sliced
2 handfuls of baby
    spinach
2 large tomatoes, cut
    into chunks
1 red onion, thinly
    sliced
oil – in a spray bottle
500 g frozen prawns,
    defrosted,
    deveined and
    washed

Dressing
juice of 2 limes
2 tbsp fish sauce
1 tbsp honey
2 cloves garlic,
    crushed

Place sliced capsicums, cucumber, spinach, tomatoes and onion in a large bowl and mix together. Set aside.

Mix all dressing ingredients together and set aside.

Heat a few pumps of oil in a wok over a high heat.

Add prawns to the wok and cook for 2–3 minutes or until cooked through.

Put prawns straight into the bowl of salad veggies, pour dressing over and serve on a large platter.

Serve it up!
• You can serve this dish on its own or with brown rice or grainy bread.

Adapt it
• Use chicken or tofu instead of prawns.

Nutrition information per serve (with dressing but without rice or bread)				
kJ = 745	Carbs = 11 g	Protein = 28 g	Fat = 2 g	Fibre = 3 g

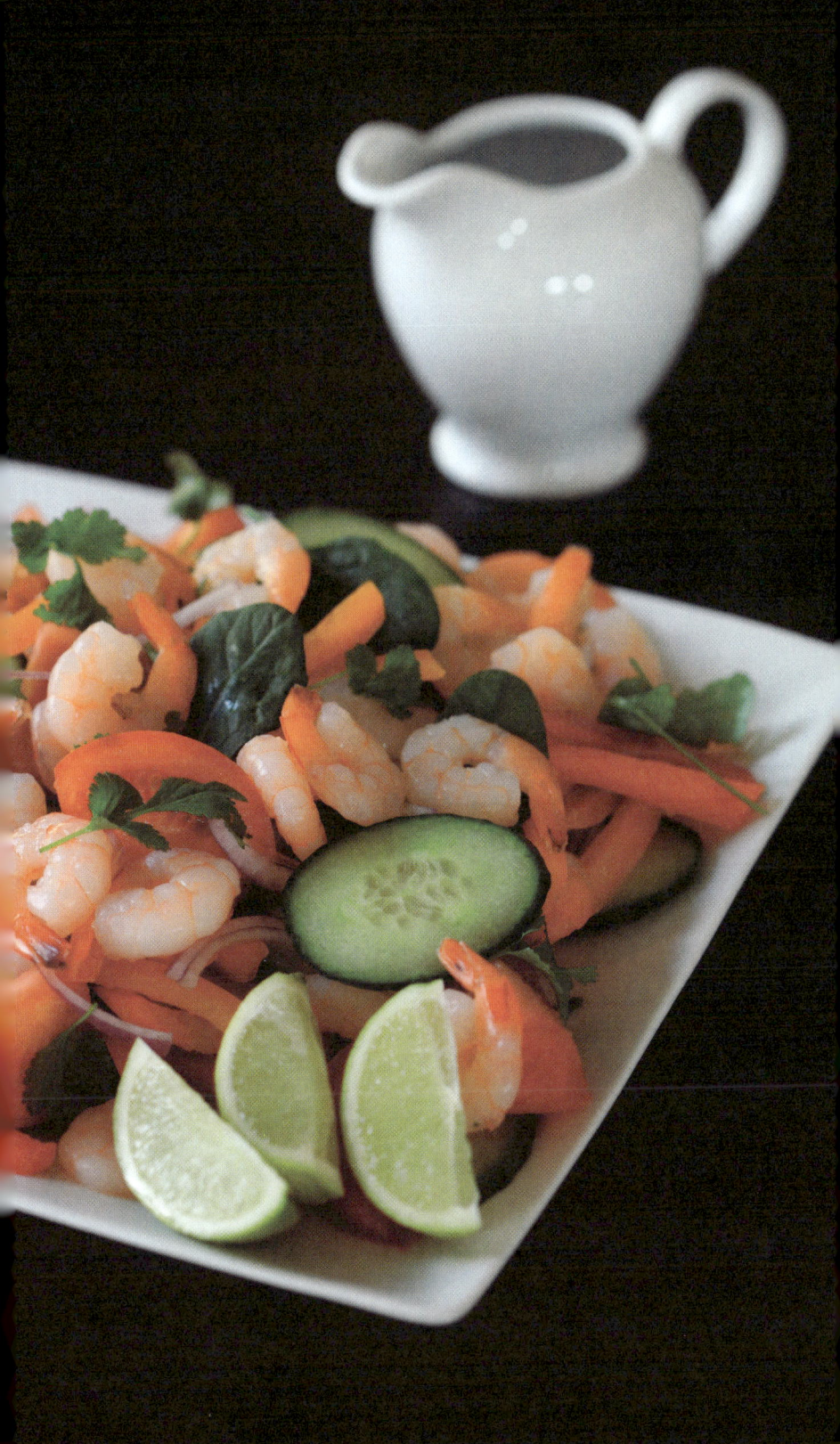

Tofu with broccoli and bulghur wheat
(Serves 2)

I have this vegetarian meal for dinner and then take the leftovers for lunch – it's nutrient-packed and delicious.

½ cup bulghur wheat
boiling water, enough to cover bulghur wheat
1 head broccoli, cut into florets
1 tsp oil
300 g tofu, chopped into chunky cubes
1 tbsp kecap manis – or sweet soy sauce
1 tbsp reduced-salt soy sauce
1 tsp sesame oil
2 tsp sesame seeds

Prepare bulghur wheat by soaking it in boiling water for 5–10 minutes. Then rinse in cold water, drain and set aside in a large bowl.

Steam broccoli florets over a saucepan of boiling water for 3–4 minutes until tender. If you don't have a steamer, cook broccoli in 1.5 cm of boiling water in a saucepan until tender and then drain. Add broccoli to bulghur wheat.

Heat oil in a non-stick frying pan, add tofu and cook for 3–4 minutes, moving it around in the pan so tofu is lightly golden on all sides.

Add kecap manis, soy sauce and sesame oil, and cook for a further minute.

Turn off the heat and sprinkle sesame seeds over.

Add tofu to steamed broccoli and bulghur wheat, and mix together.

Adapt it
• Use brown rice or quinoa instead of bulghur wheat.
• Try dressing this with the Asian dressing on page 243 – you will only need half the quantity.

Nutrition information per serve				
kJ = 1290	Carbs = 25 g	Protein = 21 g	Fat = 14 g	Fibre = 10 g

Eggplant curry *(Serves 4)*

When eggplants are in season I have this every week WITHOUT fail. It is the best vegetarian meal I have ever eaten and my husband loves it too – always a success if a man doesn't moan when there's no meat!

1 very large or
  2 medium
  eggplants
1 tsp oil
1 onion, chopped
2 tsp cumin seeds
1 tsp ground cumin
2 tsp curry powder
1 x 400 g can
  chopped
  tomatoes
1 tbsp sliced
  jalapeños – I use
  the ones in a jar
2 tbsp lite sour
  cream or natural
  yoghurt

Preheat oven to 180 °C. Line a tray with baking paper.

Place whole eggplant on the prepared tray and cook in the oven for 40 minutes or until soft. Remove from the oven and allow to cool a little.

Heat oil in a non-stick frying pan and add onion. Cook for 3–4 minutes or until brown.

Add cumin seeds, ground cumin and curry powder and cook for 2 minutes.

Carefully cut the top off the eggplant and remove all the skin.

Chop baked eggplant flesh into chunks and add to the frying pan.

Add chopped tomatoes and sliced jalapeños to the frying pan and cook for 5 minutes or until piping hot.

Stir through sour cream or yoghurt, and it's ready!

Serve it up!
- Serve with rice and any green veggies (ideally 1–2 cups per person) – beans and broccoli work really well, I find.

Nutrition information per serve (without rice or extra veggies)				
kJ = 250	Carbs = 7 g	Protein = 2 g	Fat = 3 g	Fibre = 3 g

NUTRITION INFORMATION FOR SIDES

	kJ	Carbs (g)	Protein (g)	Fat (g)	Fibre (g)
Brown rice (cooked)*					
½ cup	584	30	3	1	2
¾ cup	876	45	4	2	3
1 cup	1168	60	5	2	4
White rice (cooked)					
½ cup	448	30	2	1	1
¾ cup	672	36	3	1	1
1 cup	896	48	4	1	1
Quinoa (cooked)					
½ cup	468	20	4	2	3
¾ cup	698	30	6	3	4
1 cup	931	40	8	4	5
Pasta (cooked)					
½ cup	329	16	3	1	1
¾ cup	493	25	5	1	2
1 cup	658	33	6	1	2
Couscous (cooked)					
½ cup	326	16	4	1	1
¾ cup	488	24	5	1	2
1 cup	651	32	7	1	3
Potato (cooked)					
½ cup	280	15	2	1	1
¾ cup	419	22	3	1	2
1 cup	560	30	3	1	3
Kumara (red, cooked)					
½ cup	325	18	1	1	2
¾ cup	487	27	2	1	3
1 cup	650	37	2	1	4

* Brown rice is higher in energy per cup than white rice as it is more dense – you need a smaller serving size but it's equally filling!

	kJ	Carbs (g)	Protein (g)	Fat (g)	Fibre (g)
Lettuce					
1 cup	26	1	1	1	2
Broccoli					
1 cup	185	3	6	1	5
Spinach (steamed)					
½ cup	77	1	2	1	2
1 cup	154	3	4	1.3	4
Carrots					
1 cup	175	9	6	1	5

BOOST your veggies

It can get very dull having the same vegetables or the same basic salad every night for dinner – especially when you are trying to cover half your plate! Here are some ideas to make it more interesting.

- Grate beetroot and carrot with 1 tablespoon of lite mayo and 2 tablespoons of currants.
- Stir-fry broccoli and bokchoy with garlic, ginger and 1 teaspoon of sesame oil.
- Boil carrots in a little chicken stock with 2 teaspoons of ground ginger. Drain carrots when tender, reserving cooking stock. Boil 2 teaspoons of honey with reserved cooking stock until it thickens, then pour a little over the carrots before serving.
- Steam Savoy cabbage with green beans and courgettes. Sprinkle with chilli flakes before serving.
- Make a carrot, swede and onion mash – boil chopped vegetables together until soft, then drain and mash with ground black pepper.

To spice up vegetable sides, add any of the following:

- Stir-fried garlic, onion, ginger, fresh herbs, dried herbs – or a combination of your choice!
- Sprinkle cooked veggies with spices such as ground cumin, chilli or ground coriander.
- Add toasted pinenuts, sliced almonds or a little grated Parmesan cheese to cooked veggies.
- Chop up fresh herbs and sprinkle on cooked veggies.

SNACKS AND SWEET TREATS

I really enjoy making my own snacks and sweet treats from scratch. These are my favourite recipes for you to enjoy.

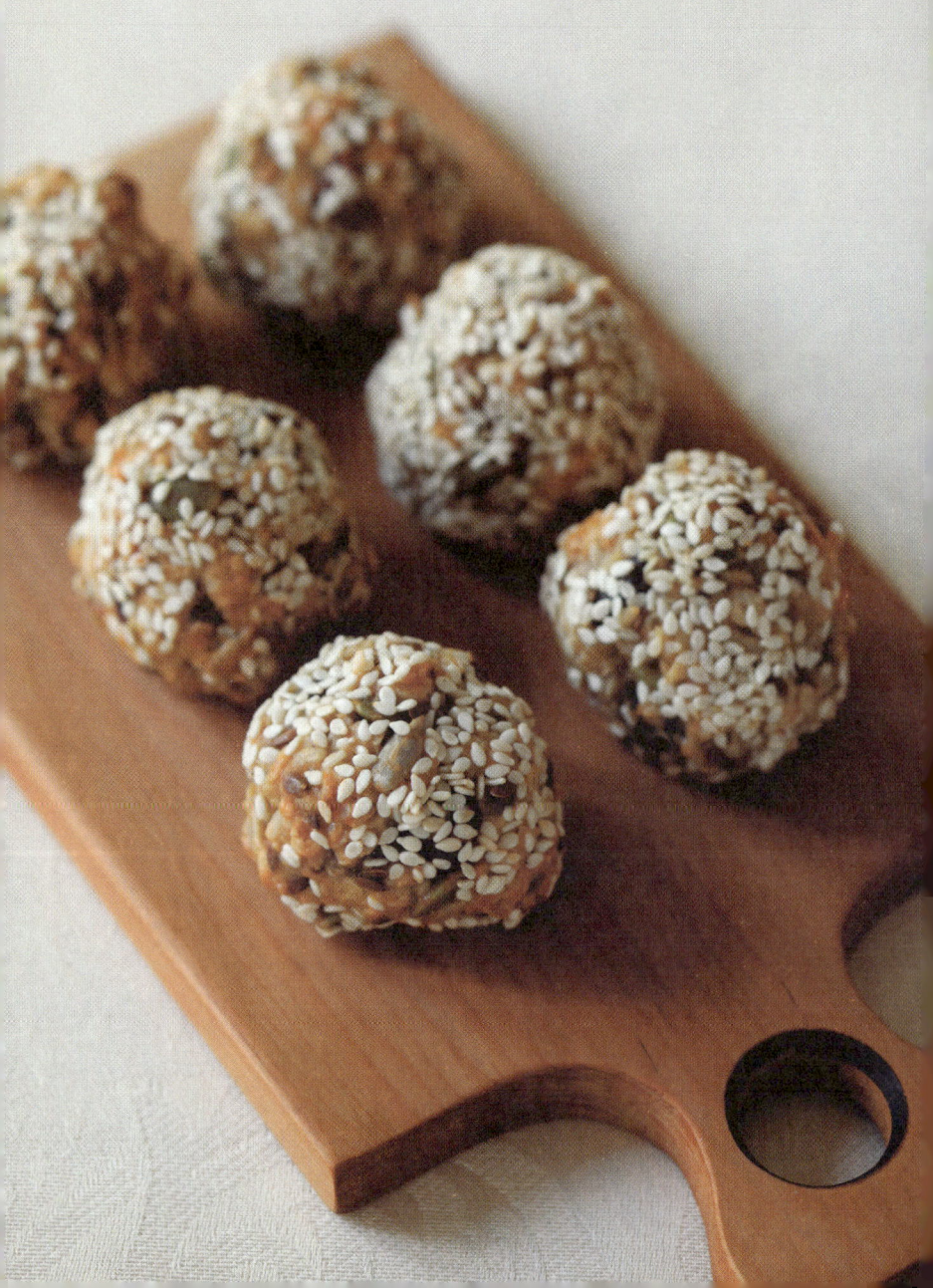

Oaty energy bites *(Makes 32)*

2 cups oats
½ cup wholemeal flour
¼ cup desiccated coconut
¼ cup sultanas
¼ cup dried cranberries
¼ cup pumpkin seeds
¼ cup sunflower seeds
2 tbsp linseeds
¼ cup chopped walnuts
⅓ cup oil
⅓ cup honey
½ cup smooth peanut butter
1 large egg, beaten
2 tbsp sesame seeds

Preheat oven to 180 °C. Line a 22 cm square baking tray with baking paper and brush lightly with oil.

Place all dry ingredients, dried fruit, seeds (apart from sesame seeds) and nuts in a bowl and mix together.

Place oil, honey and peanut butter in a saucepan and melt together over a low heat.

Pour liquid ingredients into dry ingredients and stir well.

Add egg to mixture and stir together.

Take a spoonful of mixture and roll in your hands to form a ball. Roll the ball in sesame seeds and place onto the prepared baking tray. Repeat for the rest of mixture.

Bake for 8 minutes or until golden brown.

Store in an airtight container.

Adapt it

• Swap the walnuts for hazelnuts, cashews, peanuts or any nuts you like!
• Swap linseeds for sesame seeds.

Nutrition information per bite				
kJ = 449	Carbs = 9 g	Protein = 3 g	Fat = 6 g	Fibre = 1 g

Wholesome hummus *(Serves 6)*

Hummus is SO easy to make yourself, so have a go! When you make it with yoghurt, you really need to use the hummus on the same day as it won't last. If you want a hummus to last for a day or two, check out the variations I've given below.

250 g cooked
  chickpeas
  (or 1 x 400 g
  can drained and
  rinsed)
2–3 tbsp
  unsweetened
  natural yoghurt
1 clove garlic
1 tbsp tahini –
  sesame seed paste
juice of 1 lemon
salt and ground
  black pepper
water – as needed

Simply place all the ingredients in a blender – and blend!

You may need to add more yoghurt, lemon juice or water for a smoother consistency.

Serve it up!
• Hummus is fantastic with chopped raw veggies or on wholegrain crackers with sliced tomato and black pepper – yum!

Adapt it
• Replace the yoghurt with olive oil, or try 1 tablespoon of oil and extra water – be mindful, though, that this significantly increases the kilojoule content.
• Add 2 teaspoons of ground cumin for a delicious spicy hummus.

Nutrition information per serve				
kJ = 242	Carbs = 6 g	Protein = 3 g	Fat = 3 g	Fibre = 2 g

Spicy pears with custard *(Serves 4)*

Sometimes it is nice to be able to enjoy a tasty dessert after a light meal. This is one of my favourites – the combination of flavours is just outstanding.

4 pears, peeled, cored and cut into quarters
1 tbsp honey
1 tsp cardamom
¼ tsp nutmeg – freshly grated is best
¼ tsp ground cinnamon
¼ cup water
2 cups custard (made with low-fat milk)
10 walnuts, chopped

Place pears in a saucepan with honey, spices and water.

Simmer gently for around 10 minutes, then leave to cool.

Divide pears into small bowls or glass dishes and top with ½ cup of custard each. Scatter walnuts over each dish.

Adapt it

- Serve this hot or cold: either cool the pears and serve with chilled custard or serve the pears warm with hot custard.
- Replace the water with a sweet dessert wine for special occasions.
- Serve the pears hot or cold with low-fat yoghurt instead of custard in summer.

Nutrition information per serve				
kJ = 1183	Carbs = 42 g	Protein = 9 g	Fat = 9 g	Fibre = 3 g

Banana bran muffins *(Makes 12 muffins)*

These are a good snack and they freeze well, too!

2 cups oat bran
½ cup wholemeal flour
1 tsp baking powder
1 tsp baking soda
1 tsp ground cinnamon
½ cup sultanas
2 medium-sized ripe bananas, mashed
1 egg, beaten
1 cup trim milk
½ cup golden syrup or honey

Preheat oven to 180 °C. Lightly spray oil onto a 12-hole muffin tray.

Place all dry ingredients and sultanas in a bowl.

Add mashed bananas to dry ingredients.

Add egg, milk and syrup or honey and stir well.

Spoon mixture into the prepared trays.

Bake for 10–12 minutes or until golden brown and springy to the touch. Remove from oven and cool in the tray before turning out.

Nutrition information per serve				
kJ = 747	Carbs = 35 g	Protein = 5 g	Fat = 2 g	Fibre = 4 g

Berry breeze *(Serves 1)*

This is a delicious treat which is mainly fruit!

¾ cup frozen blueberries or raspberries
1 pottle (150 g) low-fat berry yoghurt – or unsweetened if you prefer
1 tsp berry jam

Place all ingredients in a blender and blitz together to make a frozen fruity dessert.

Adapt it
• If you prefer a softer texture, add a splash of milk.

Nutrition information per serve				
kJ = 572	Carbs = 26 g	Protein = 7 g	Fat = <1 g	Fibre = 2 g

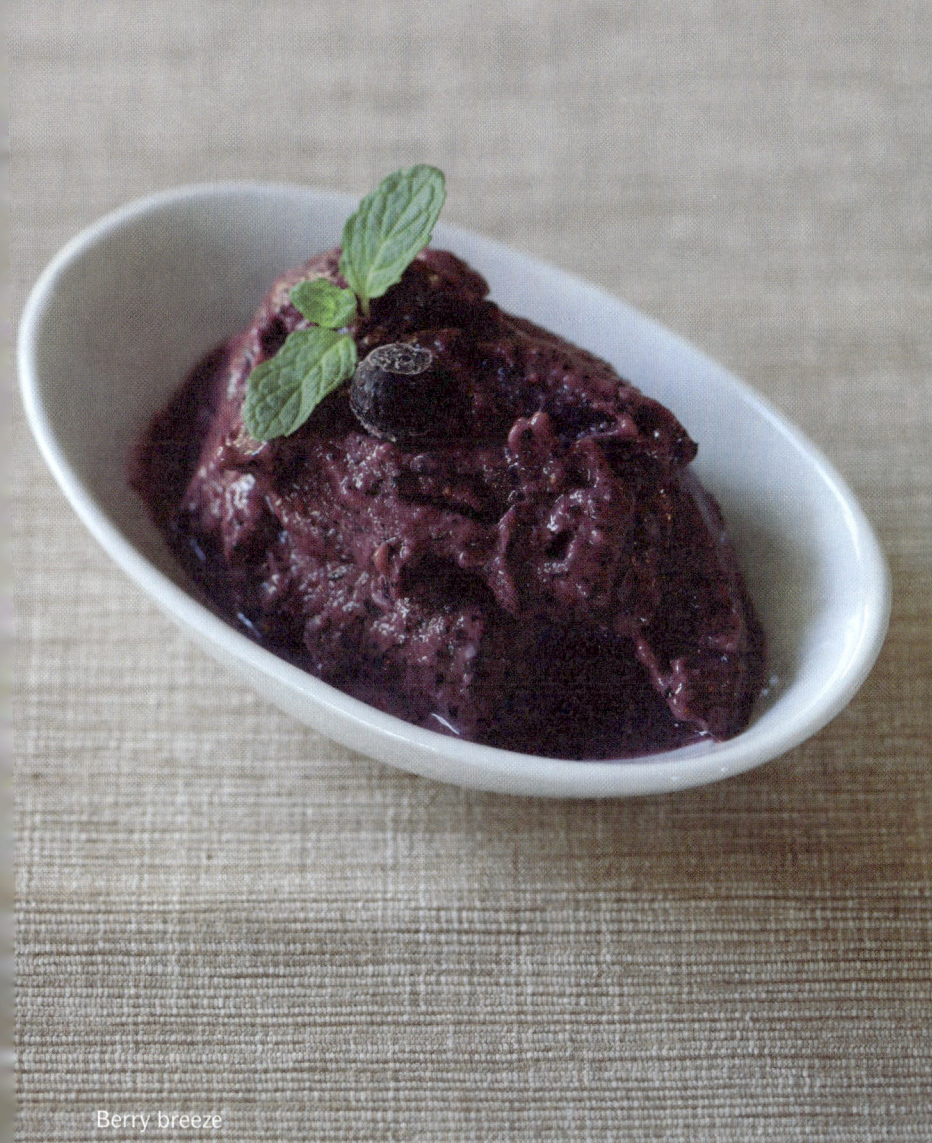
Berry breeze

References and Resources

Bender, David A. *Introduction to Nutrition and Metabolism*, second edition, Taylor & Francis, London, 1997.

Ford, Debbie. *The Right Questions: Ten Essential Questions to Guide You to an Extraordinary Life*, Harper San Francisco, San Francisco, 2004.

Ministry of Health. Food and Nutrition Guidelines for Healthy Adults: A Background Paper, Ministry of Health, Wellington, 2003. Available at: http://www.health.govt.nz/publication/food-and-nutrition-guidelines-healthy-adults-background-paper.

National Health and Medical Research Council (NHMRC). Nutrient Reference Values for Australia and New Zealand Including Recommended Dietary Intakes. Available at: http://www.nrv.gov.au/nutrients/index.htm.

Tortora, Gerard J. and Bryan Derrickson. *Principles of Anatomy and Physiology*, twelfth edition, John Wiley & Sons, Inc., 2009.

University of Otago and Ministry of Health. A Focus on Nutrition: Key Findings of the 2008/09 New Zealand Adult Nutrition Survey. Ministry of Health, Wellington, 2011. Available at: http://www.health.govt.nz/publication/focus-nutrition-key-findings-2008-09-nz-adult-nutrition-survey.

Wansink, Brian. *Mindless Eating: Why We Eat More Than We Think*, Bantam Books, New York, 2010.

WEBSITES

Alcohol Advisory Council of New Zealand – www.alac.org.nz
CSIRO – www.csiro.au
Foodworks 2009 – http://www.xyris.com.au/foodworks/download.html
Heart Foundation – www.heartfoundation.co.nz
Kidney Health New Zealand www.kidneys.co.nz
Omega-3 Centre – www.omega-3centre.com

OTHER USEFUL WEBSITES

Dr Alex Bartle (Sleep Specialist) – www.sleepwellclinic.co.nz
Claire Turnbull – www.claireturnbull.co.nz
Dave Margison (Personal Trainer) – www.workout.co.nz
Healthy Food Guide – www.healthyfood.co.nz
Dr Joanna McMillan (Dietitian and Vice President of the Australian Lifestyle Medicine Association) – www.drjoanna.com.au
Jenny Devine (Integrative Coach) – www.jennydevine.co.nz
Louise Thompson (Life Coach and Yoga Instructor) – www.positivebalance.co.nz
Mission Nutrition (Dietitians and Nutritionists) – www.missionnutrition.co.nz

Thanks and Acknowledgements

First, I would like to acknowledge those who have helped me to put this book together and to make it magic.

Louise Thompson, you are an amazing woman with incredible wisdom. You have helped me to understand the power of our thoughts and that we can all achieve anything we dream of. Thanks for your help, love and support – look forward to continuing to work with you and changing the world. Dr Alex Bartle, thank you for opening my eyes to the value of rest, recovery and a good night's sleep as part of living a balanced healthy life. Dave Margison, thanks for kicking my arse at the gym and sharing your knowledge with your fitness programmes. Jenny Devine, you have opened my eyes to a world of 'being', taking 100 per cent responsibility for your life and a daily commitment to not making things right or wrong – I am so glad I met you and love working with you. Dr Joanna McMillan, thanks for reviewing my work and for supporting what I am doing. You are awesome and I totally admire your commitment to and passion for the work you do.

Second, I would like to acknowledge those who have worked with me, supported and encouraged me to get to a point where I could even consider writing a book. Denis Snelgar, for your incredible insight, vision and unquestionable faith in me, thank you. Craig Jones and Kim Mundell, without you both I wouldn't have ever had the courage to go out on my own and work for myself – thanks for believing in me. To Diabetes Auckland, thanks for giving me my first job in New Zealand which allowed me to discover this amazing country and eventually set up my life here.

Third, and by no means last, to my friends and family who have always believed in me, who have encouraged me and without fail love me to the ends of the earth. Mum and Dad, you are amazing and have taught me to always do my best. I love you and hope to make you proud with everything I do. To my brothers James and Luke, thanks for teaching me a lot about myself when we were growing up, and thanks also for your encouragement and love ever since. To my incredible husband who unconditionally stands by me and has helped me be the best I can be, thank you – I couldn't have done any of this without your love and support. To my fabulous friends – you know who you are – thanks for not giving up on me in hard times; without you I wouldn't be here to share my story, knowledge and experiences. I am so blessed and lucky to have you all.

To my staff at Mission Nutrition, the team at *Healthy Food Guide* magazine and everyone I have met along the way so far on my journey in health and wellness – you have made it clear to me that I am doing the right thing with my life and you help keep my inspiration and passion alive.

Thanks, of course, to you for taking the time to read this book. I hope it helps you to be the best you can be. I also hope this book helps you realise that you are absolutely amazing. You need to learn to love yourself for who you are and, most importantly, that life is there for living.

Claire Turnbull

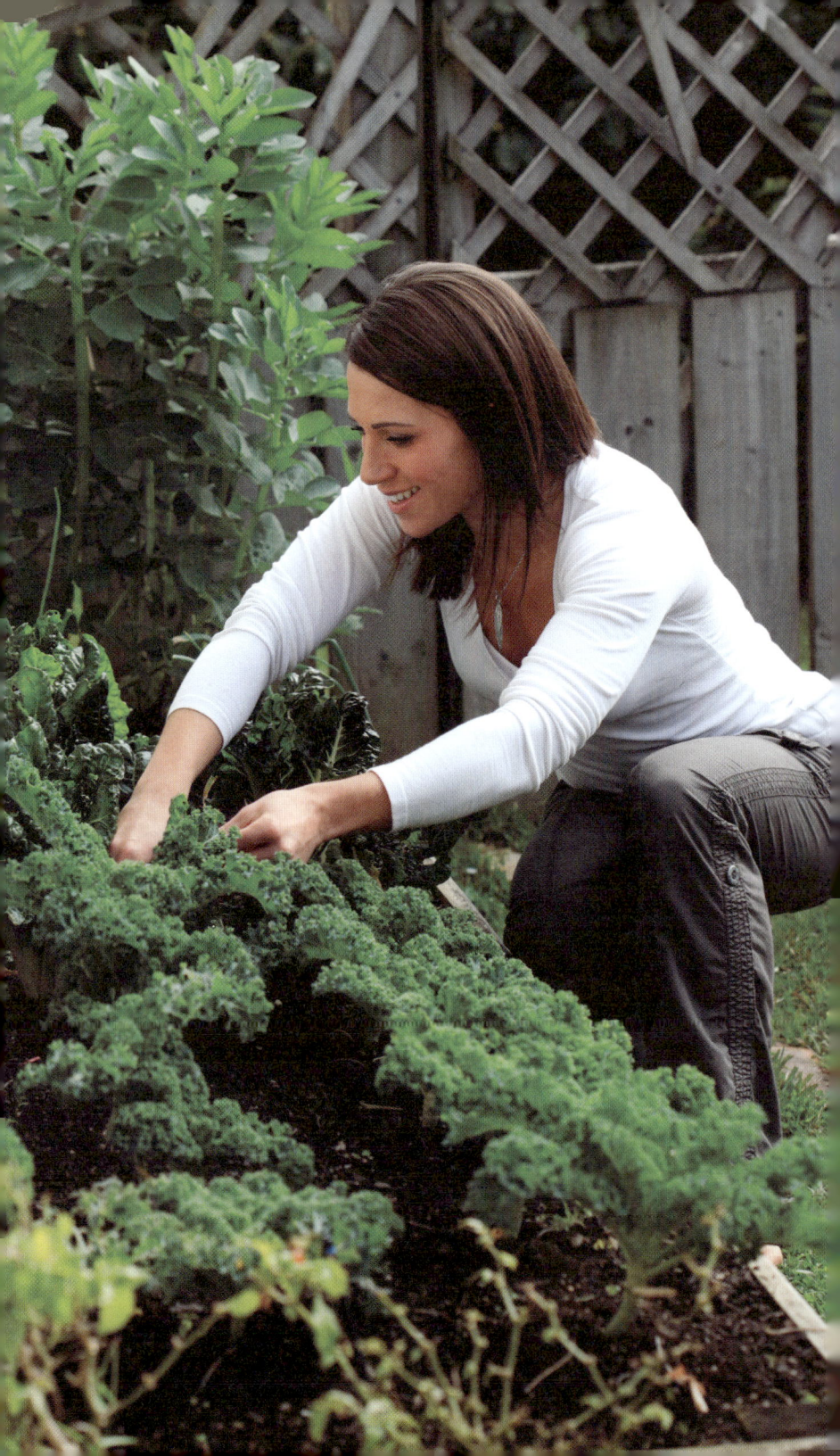

Index

Recipes index

A

B